"Nicole Doña has written *The Mind-Spirit Bible Practice* bridging the concepts of Dialectical Behavior Therapy with Biblical Spirituality—two worlds that are often kept separate but are deeply complementary. Doña thoughtfully laid out how DBT skills like mindfulness, emotion regulation, and distress tolerance can be lived both clinically and spiritually. Written with candor and vulnerability, *The Mind-Spirit Bible Practice* is relatable for those facing emotional or mental health challenges, the stigma of diagnosis and spiritual dissonance that so often accompanies these experiences."

—Tessa Kwan,
Licensed Marriage & Family Therapist

"I was deeply moved by Doña's life story and her ability to navigate profound hardship with honesty and grace. Many people might become weary, hardened, or cynical in the face of so much pain, but Doña shows what it looks like to put Dialectical Behavior Therapy into practice alongside meditation on Scripture—transforming suffering into strength, wisdom, and fortitude.

Reading this book felt like savoring a rich chocolate cake—so full, layered, and satisfying that you want to slow down and take your time with it. Each chapter invites reflection, allowing the truths to sink in rather than be rushed past. Doña's vulnerability gave me faith and hope in my own journey, along with a gentle but powerful pathway toward healing. I believe anyone who takes the time to truly sit with this book will find it deeply sustaining and transformative."

—Jennifer Larsen,
House Church Leader

"For those of you who are stuck and seeking a way out, I highly recommend *The Mind-Spirit Bible Practice* as a place to start. Nicole Doña blesses us with her moving testimony of healing and wholeness, meeting readers with compassion and honesty right where they are. This book aligns biblical wisdom principles with DBT stepping stones that light the way toward integrating mind, body, and spirit. I believe it can be especially valuable when used alongside therapy or within ministry settings, offering a shared, trauma-informed language that supports both personal reflection and guided care."

—Dayne Bartlett, MSW, LICSW, LADC,
Founder of Create Meaning LLC

The Mind–Spirit Bible Practice

A Trauma-Informed DBT Inspired
Guide to Renew the Mind & Spirit

NICOLE DOÑA

LUCIDBOOKS

The Mind-Spirit Bible Practice: A Trauma-Informed DBT Inspired Guide to Renew the Mind & Spirit

Published by Lucid Books in Houston, TX
www.LucidBooks.com

ISBN: 978-1-63296-977-4
eISBN: 978-1-63296-978-1

Disclaimer

The views, interpretations, and applications expressed in this book are solely those of the author. They do not reflect the views or positions of any current or former employer, affiliated organization, public agency, faith-based or other institution.

References to Dialectical Behavior Therapy (DBT) are for educational and integrative purposes only. This book is not affiliated with, endorsed by, or sponsored by Marsha M. Linehan, PhD, ABPP; Behavioral Tech, LLC; or any DBT certifying body.

The Mind–Spirit Bible Practice is an independent framework developed by the author and is not an official or certified DBT model.

Dedication

To my mother, Jacqueline Plata, who never gives up, models resilience, and challenges me to pursue my dreams. And to my husband, Joshua Doña, my partner in bringing those dreams to life and keeping me grounded along the way. I love you both.

Contents

Part I
From the Divided Mind to
the Renewed Integrated Mind

Part II
The Practice: Living from the Mind of the Spirit

A Note to the Reader

This book was written at the intersection of faith and mental health—a space that is both tender and holy. As you read, you may find your heart stirred, your memories awakened, or your body responding in ways you didn't expect. That is normal. Healing is holy work, and sometimes healing feels like trembling.

This book is not meant to be rushed. Some chapters may feel immediately familiar; others may surface resistance, grief, or conviction. That, too, is part of the work. You may find it helpful to read slowly, return to certain sections, journal, or reflect alongside a trusted friend, therapist, pastor, or spiritual community.

This book is not a replacement for therapy, nor is it a shortcut to spiritual maturity. It is an invitation to integration—to notice where your inner life, your relationships, and your faith are being gently brought under the loving rule of God. Take what meets you where you are, and trust that God will meet you there too.

Objectives of This Book

The goal of *The Mind–Spirit Bible Practice* is to build a bridge between evidence-based psychology and Christian spiritual formation. Drawing from Dialectical Behavior Therapy (DBT) and Scripture, this book explores how clinical tools can be illuminated and deepened through the wisdom of God's Word—supporting growth in emotional regulation, resilience, and spiritual maturity.

This book is written for Christians seeking to understand their emotional and mental life through a biblical lens, as well as for clinicians, pastors, and ministry leaders who desire to engage faith as a meaningful ally in the healing process. Each chapter offers a framework that integrates psychological skill with spiritual wisdom—not for self-improvement, but for transformation through the renewing work of the Holy Spirit.

This book is meant to be a companion, not a substitute for professional care. It is written for those already walking a path of healing—through counseling, prayer, community, or quiet perseverance. If you encounter a section that stirs pain too heavy to carry alone, that is not a sign of weakness; it is a sign that something important within you is asking for care. Bring it to a trusted counselor, pastor, mentor, or friend.

As you read, give yourself permission to pause. Take a breath. Pray a verse aloud. Notice where your body holds peace or tension. Invite the Holy Spirit to meet you there.

This book tells my story—the way I experienced it, the way it shaped me, and the way God continues to redeem it. Some sections touch on trauma, family complexity, or community violence. These moments are shared not to assign blame or expose anyone's private life, but to bear honest witness to God's healing presence. Wherever appropriate, names and identifying details have been changed to protect privacy.

My intention is not to tell other people's stories, but to tell my own—through the lens of grace and growth. The people who appear in these pages are complex and human, just as I am. Many did the best they could with what they had.

I believe every story—even those marked by suffering—can become a place where God's love is revealed. My prayer is that as you read mine, you sense the same presence that met me in my brokenness: the God who fills every gap with mercy, wholeness, and hope.

With love and reverence,
Nicole Doña

Author's Note
on Scope & Integration

This book was written at the intersection of faith, emotional life, and lived experience. It draws from my personal story, years of spiritual formation, and engagement with evidence-based psychological concepts—particularly Dialectical Behavior Therapy (DBT)—as tools that helped me remain present with God in seasons of distress, healing, and growth.

This book is **not a clinical manual**, nor is it intended to diagnose, treat, or replace professional mental-health care. I am not writing as a clinician, but as a practitioner of faith who has benefited deeply from therapy, medication, spiritual direction, and community. Where psychological language appears, it is used to *illuminate experience*, not to prescribe treatment.

The practices in these pages are offered as **spiritual formation**, not psychological intervention. They are meant to help readers notice their inner life, cultivate awareness, tolerate distress without shame, and return—again and again—to the presence of God. Scripture remains the primary authority and lens of this book; psychological frameworks serve as companions, not replacements, for that work.

Readers are encouraged to engage this book slowly, prayerfully, and in discernment with their own support systems. For some, that may include therapy, pastoral care, spiritual direction, or trusted community. If at any point the material brings up pain that feels too heavy to carry alone, that is not a failure of faith—it is an invitation to seek wise and compassionate support.

My hope is not that readers would become more skilled at managing themselves, but more rooted in God's presence. Integration, as I use the term, is not about mastery or control—it is about learning to remain with God in the truth of our humanity, trusting that He meets us there with grace, wisdom, and love.

Finding Wholeness in the Gap

"I searched for someone who would repair the wall, one who fills the gap, an intercessor to cry out for mercy, but I found no one . . ."

—Ezekiel 22:30 (TPT)

"Therefore He [Jesus] is able also to save forever (completely, perfectly, for eternity) those who come to God through Him, since He always lives to intercede and intervene on their behalf [with God]."

—Hebrews 7:25 (AMP)

I've spent most of my life trying to fix what I didn't understand needed holy integration.

I used to think healing meant never breaking again.

Now I know it means learning how to keep searching for God in the cracks.

If you've ever wondered whether faith and psychology can coexist—or if your emotions disqualify you from God's peace—this book is for you.

There's a reason I'm still standing.

This book isn't just about the pain, trauma, and sin that broke me—it's about the God who keeps rebuilding me. It's about learning, and re-learning, how to wholly walk with God in a world that keeps fracturing us daily.

Somewhere along the way, I also had to unlearn something deeply damaging: the idea that everything that happens is God's will. Scripture never asks us to believe that abuse, neglect, or harm are authored by God. Jesus does not explain suffering away—He moves toward it. God's will, as revealed in Christ, is not control over every outcome, but communion within every moment. That distinction matters—especially for those of us whose stories, like mine, include trauma.

My story begins in chaos, but somewhere in the middle of it, I began to see a hunger for connection—with God, which ultimately and slowly helped heal the disconnect within myself, and with others.

I didn't always know how to bridge these gaps. For most of my life, I felt like a walking contradiction—loved and unwanted, gifted and misunderstood, too much and never enough. I still feel that way sometimes, a lot of the time. But the longer I walk with Jesus, the more I see how He steps into every disconnect, to meet me there, to intercede for me, and bring me into God's presence. As Jesus teaches me to walk with Him, He is integrating every part of my life with meaning, healing, and grace.

That's what the Mind Spirit Bible Practice (MSB) is about. It's the framework that grew from my story—an integration of faith, emotion, and the mind of Christ. It's the bridge I searched for between my therapy sessions and my prayer life, between my diagnoses and my discipleship, between my trauma and God's justice, between modern psychology and Biblical wisdom. I didn't invent it; it always existed—it was revealed to me over many years of tension, wrestling, doubting, learning, and realizing that healing isn't found in choosing between the two, but in letting faith and psychology work together.

The goal of this book is to create a bridge between evidence-based psychology and Christian spiritual formation, to help those of us who suffer find courage and tools to enter into a life filled with God's presence, building confidence without shame and with full assurance of the mercy and grace found through Christ. It's written for both Christians who long to understand their emotions through a biblical lens and for clinicians, pastors, and ministry leaders who wish to engage faith as a meaningful ally in the healing process for those in our communities who feel they are too far gone. The Mind Spirit Bible Practice invites readers to explore how the tools of Dialectical Behavior Therapy (DBT) can be illuminated and deepened through Scripture, helping individuals grow in emotional regulation, resilience, and spiritual maturity to fully experience the Kingdom of Heaven on earth.

Each chapter offers a framework that integrates clinical skill with spiritual wisdom—inviting readers to move beyond self-improvement, toward transformation, through the renewing work of the Holy Spirit, allowing us to live our lives filled with God's presence. My prayer is that through this integration, you'll discover not only how to manage emotions but how to meet God within them—learning to live, as Romans 8:6 says, "from the mind governed by the Spirit," which brings life and peace.

Early on in elementary school, teachers said I was unruly but oddly bright. "She's never listening," they'd tell my mom, "but she always seems to know the answer."

Attempting to put me on the spot, my teachers would call me to the board to be tested, but I'd solve the problem in seconds. One teacher wrote on my report card, "She's disruptive, but always seems to have one ear listening."

Every year, I was referred to the GATE Program—Gifted and Talented Education—but I never passed the standardized test. I'd watch the GATE students leave for their "special" classes and wonder what they were learning. So when I was pulled out of class for what I didn't know at the time was therapy, I thought maybe I was "just too smart" to be in class. I got to play and talk about my life while everyone else was stuck doing classwork. Therapy just felt like playtime.

It wasn't until years later, at twenty-two, when I began processing my trauma, that I realized what those sessions really were. They were, in fact, play therapy, and it was evident so early on that my mental health and trauma responses were shaping how I interacted with the world—and how the world interacted with me.

Now, looking back, I can see it: even then, God was planting the seeds that would evolve into MSB—long before I knew I'd need them to survive. Not because God caused the harm I endured, but because He never stopped working toward healing in the midst of it.

I always felt different.

I'm biracial—Puerto Rican and Panamanian on my mom's side, Caucasian on my father's. I grew up in East San Jose, California, surrounded by gang culture, addiction, and poverty—yet my parents worked in Silicon Valley as engineers and managers at tech companies.

I was "too smart" for regular classes but never quite smart enough for GATE. Too White for some, too Latina for others. I didn't speak Spanish (yet) and didn't fit the mold of any culture I belonged to. By the time I was twelve, I had lived through four divorces between my parents, endured many forms of abuse—physical, emotional, and sexual— been confronted with community-based violence, and felt utterly alone.

At the time, I thought my differences were proof that I didn't belong anywhere. Learning to bridge the polarities in my identity has been my training ground. My complexity—the ache of not fitting in, the constant pull between extremes—became the very thing that helped me grasp the divide between Christianity and Psychology. It taught me to hold tension, to live in paradox.

The same dialectical pull that defined my life—being both spiritual and emotional, logical and passionate, strong and broken—became the same tension that now defines my continued healing in Christ.

I didn't know how to cope. I was bored and angry.

At twelve years old, my world already felt loud and unsafe. My mom and I had just moved out of my stepdad's house, my older brother was incarcerated for dealing drugs, and my father had moved back to Illinois. All the men who had once made me feel safe and loved were suddenly gone.

My mom worked long hours to support us—leaving early each morning while I woke up alone, got myself ready, and walked to school.

On those walks, older men would catcall me. I'd cross the street to avoid drug dealers. I learned to look "hard," to make myself seem unapproachable, even though I felt anything but. I was on high alert and hypervigilant all the time. I looked too "White" to blend in and wasn't a fighter, so I learned early to read a room before I entered it—to sense tension, to stay big and act too tough to mess with. Everyone at school was doing the same—trying to look strong enough to survive.

I started sneaking boys into my mom's house—engaging in sexual activities no twelve-year-old should be doing— experimenting with substances, and at thirteen, I was arrested at school in front of all my friends. The shame was unbearable. I was shunned by my peers, mocked, and left to navigate my depression and anxiety in silence. Shame became my language. I pushed people away before they could reject me.

Looking back now, I understand with compassion that much of my childhood unfolded outside the safety, order, and protection of God's will and Kingdom—not because God was absent, but because His presence was resisted, ignored, or unavailable in the world around me.

My father had taken me to church when I was small, but my mom and stepdad did not practice any religion. By this point, I had already decided God must be cruel—if He even existed at all.

Then one day, one of my mom's friends invited us to church. I'd sit in the back row with crossed arms, scowling, refusing to participate or speak to anyone. But another teenage girl from the youth group walked up and introduced herself. She invited herself over to my house, shared her story, and told me how she read her Bible daily for comfort and guidance.

Her persistence annoyed me—but it also intrigued me. Out of boredom, I decided to open the Bible for myself. I was very curious, so I began reading the Book of Revelation, and then I found this verse:

"For the Lamb at the center of the throne will be
their shepherd;
He will lead them to springs of living water.
And God will wipe away every tear from their eyes."
(Revelation 7:17)

That verse changed everything—or maybe it just started something.

For years, I hadn't cried. I didn't think anyone cared about my tears. But this verse said otherwise—that God Himself noticed them, cared about them, and would wipe each one away.

If that kind of God was real, I wanted to know Him.

At fourteen, I began devouring the Bible. I read it before school, at lunch, and before bed. I had finally found a love that could hold my pain and my internal chaos—but it didn't make them disappear. It just meant I didn't have to face them all alone anymore. Even then, I didn't realize I was being led to those same springs of living water Revelation spoke of—and that I'd spend years learning how to trust and believe it was safe to drink from them.

So many life-changing miracles followed that decision—but despite the miracles, that decision didn't make life easy.

I faced seasons that broke me open again and again— being diagnosed with complex PTSD, bipolar disorder, and borderline personality disorder. I learned I had a brain tumor that paralyzed one of my vocal cords, and I had an implant to help me speak. I had surgeries that didn't always work and moments when my own body felt like a battlefield. Despite all this, I graduated from college with honors. I married a gentle, faithful man. I built a career I love, started a nonprofit organization, and became a foster mom.

And yet—every one of those moments became an invitation to return to God's presence, through His Word, to find comfort, validation, guidance, and sometimes just for survival. Each time life knocked me down, Jesus met me there in my brokenness. When I couldn't speak, the Holy Spirit prayed for me. When I couldn't regulate my emotions, His Word steadied me. When I wanted to quit, His grace caught me.

Healing wasn't linear. It still isn't. It's costly, slow, and sacred.

Through all of this, I've learned that psychology and psychiatry are tools, but not the *source* of healing. Ecclesiastes 10:10 says, "If the ax is dull and its edge unsharpened, more strength is needed, but skill will bring success."

Therapy and medication sharpen the ax, but only God's presence gives the strength to use it. Therapy taught me how to cope, but the Spirit teaches me God's purpose and calling, and gives me the motivation to keep going.

This is where the MSB practice was born—not from triumph, but from tension. Out of the realization that faith and psychology were never meant to be rivals. Together, they reveal a fuller picture of healing:

- **Mindfulness** becomes being present in God's presence.
- **Distress tolerance** becomes sitting in the wilderness with God.

- **Emotion regulation** becomes letting the Spirit rule the heart.

- **Interpersonal effectiveness** becomes speaking the truth in love.

That's redemption. That's what God does—He not only integrates what was once fragmented, He shows us how, by the Divine coming in a human form—Jesus.

Matthew 1:22-23 (TPT) says, "This happened to fulfill what the Lord had spoken through his prophet: Listen! A virgin will be pregnant, she will give birth to a Son, and he will be known as "Emmanuel," which means in Hebrew, "God became one of us.""

God integrates the supernatural, the spiritual, and the eternal with the natural, the flesh, and humanity. Jesus is the case study by which we learn how to live integrated lives as spiritual human beings, living in a broken world and seeking and living out His Kingdom.

When I look back, I can see the spiritual and human thread running through it all: the girl who once needed play therapy now advocates for children living her story. The one who thought she'd never belong now builds communities of belonging. The woman who felt she was too broken to mother now mothers children whose trauma mirrors her own.

Paul writes in his letter to the Corinthians:

We are like common clay jars that carry this glorious treasure within, so that this immeasurable power will be seen as God's, not ours. Though we experience every kind of pressure, we're not crushed. At times we don't know what to do, but quitting is not an option. We are persecuted by others, but God has not forsaken us. We may be knocked down, but not out. We continually share in the death of Jesus in our own bodies so that the resurrection life of Jesus will be revealed through our humanity. (2 Corinthians 4:7-10 TPT)

The brokenness I feel is human, and every day I still wrestle with it—with my shame, my guilt, my sin, my trauma, my limits. I still fall apart, but I found that Jesus's supernatural spiritual power transported me into God's presence and infused Himself into my mind, my body, and my humanity every time I opened my Bible and prayed.

God never intended my pain, but my pain has never been wasted. God's goodness keeps turning every season of suffering into a source of empathy and every failure into an opportunity to see His grace more clearly. He's taken what once felt like disconnection and turned it into the foundation for deeper connection—with Him, with others, and with myself.

I'm not writing this because I've figured it all out.

I'm writing this because I haven't—but I've found the One who stands in the gap when I can't.

If not for the consistent return to God's Word since I was fourteen, I believe I'd be lost in darkness. Jesus keeps standing in the gap for me—repairing years of rejection, trauma, sin, and isolation—and building a bridge of faith, hope, love, and the supernatural power of His Kingdom that still holds me today.

This is a story about finding God in the gap—between our fallen world and the glory of who He's calling us to be in His Kingdom. Not just for your own healing, but so others can find hope too. It's about discovering that even when everything falls apart, He's already there, rebuilding something more beautiful than before.

If He could stand in the gap for me, He can do the same for you.

And He will—even if it takes a lifetime to believe it.

In the chapters ahead, I'll share how this discovery—the Mind Spirit Bible Practice—grew into a way of life, a way of walking with Jesus, a way of healing, a way of seeing Jesus as the ultimate model of integration between mind, emotion, and Spirit, and a way to find God's Kingdom.

This book is written for anyone who's ever felt torn between their faith and their feelings, and anyone tired of feeling like a victim of their pain, trauma, and suffering. This is for believers seeking victory, and even clinicians who long to understand how Biblical spirituality and psychology can be reconciled.

As you read these pages, you may notice a rhythm that moves from the personal to the communal. This book began as my search for peace in the tension between faith and emotion, but what I found was God's presence and His Kingdom. Healing never stays private for long, nor is it meant to. This is a call to those who are seeking the same God who integrates the divided mind and gathers His people into one Body—His Kingdom—so that none of us heals alone.

My hope is that by the final chapter, you will see how the skills we practice individually—awareness, compassion, regulation, truth in love—become the lifeblood of the culture in God's Kingdom. The Spirit who steadies us in solitude is the same Spirit who unites us at the banquet table. My wholeness did not begin with me and was never meant to end with me; it was meant to be multiplied through *us*.

A Simple Overview of Dialectical Behavior Therapy

Disclaimer

The following overview is for educational and inspirational purposes only and to provide a brief background into DBT to set the stage for the rest of my book. I am not a licensed clinician or a DBT-certified provider. My goal is simply to introduce the core ideas of Dialectical Behavior Therapy (DBT) and to show how its practical wisdom mirrors many biblical truths about emotional growth, grace, and transformation. If you wish to study or practice DBT clinically, please seek guidance from a licensed mental-health professional trained in DBT.

What Is DBT?

Dialectical Behavior Therapy—often called DBT—was developed by psychologist Dr. Marsha Linehan in 1993 to help people who experience emotions very strongly (Linehan 2015). The word *dialectical* means that two ideas that seem opposite can both be true at the same time—for example, *"I'm doing my best, and I want to do better"* (Linehan 2015). Dialectics is just another way of saying a "paradox" which is widely accepted in the Christian faith.

DBT teaches practical life skills for handling big emotions, building healthy relationships (Koerner 2012), and making choices that reflect our deepest values. Over time, it has become one of the most effective evidence-based therapies for emotional regulation, trauma recovery, and relationship repair (Stoffers et al. 2012).

The Four Core Skill Areas

DBT organizes its tools into four main modules—Mindfulness, Distress Tolerance, Emotion Regulation, and Interpersonal Effectiveness (Linehan 2015). Each one addresses a key part of what it means to live wisely and well. Together, they form a balanced foundation for emotional growth.

1. Mindfulness

What It Encompasses

Mindfulness means "paying attention, on purpose, in the present moment, without judgment" (Kabat-Zinn 1994)

In DBT, mindfulness includes "what" skills (observe, describe, participate) and "how" skills (non-judgmentally, one-mindfully, effectively) (Linehan 2015).

How It Helps

Mindfulness slows the racing mind and lets us notice what's happening before we react (Soler et al. 2012). It creates space for wiser choices and greater peace. Spiritually, mindfulness deepens our awareness of God's presence in each moment (Willard 1998).

How It's Practiced

Mindfulness begins where awareness meets grace. It starts with a pause—a sacred breath between impulse and intention.

In DBT, this looks like learning to observe what's happening, to describe it honestly (Linehan 2015), and to participate in the moment as it is, not as we wish it were.

It's less about emptying the mind and more about *anchoring* it—to truth, to presence, to God's steadying love.

Wise Mind:
The Integration of Truth and Emotion

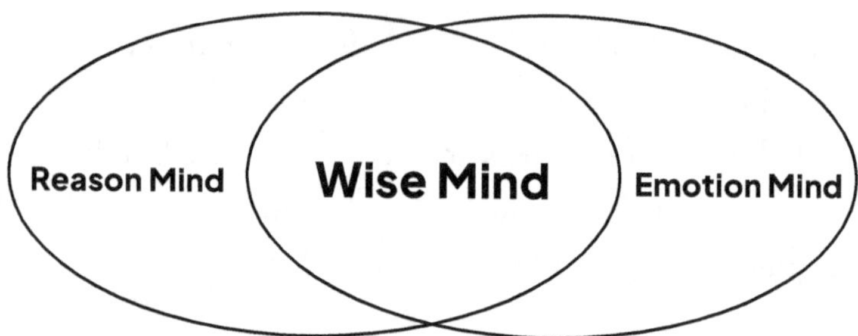

At the heart of DBT's mindfulness teaching is something called the Wise Mind—the inner meeting place between Emotion Mind and Reason Mind (Linehan 2015).

- Emotion Mind is driven by what we *feel* in the moment—passion, pain, fear, or joy. It's powerful, but it can sweep us away if we let it steer alone.

- Reason Mind is guided by logic and facts. It helps us plan, analyze, and think clearly, but without emotion, it can feel cold or disconnected.

- Wise Mind is where the two meet—a balanced awareness that honors both truth and feeling. It's the quiet center where clarity and compassion coexist.

When we live from Wise Mind, we respond instead of reacting. We pause long enough to sense what's true and what's loving. In Scripture, this aligns beautifully with the "mind governed by the Spirit" (Romans 8:6)—where truth and grace no longer compete, but work together in harmony.

Over time, Wise Mind becomes not just a DBT concept but a spiritual posture—a way of walking through life attentive to both wisdom and love, head and heart, truth and grace.

Biblical Parallel

"Be still, and know that I am God" (Psalm 46:10).

Mindfulness echoes the ancient discipline of stillness—listening for God in the present moment and aligning the mind with His Spirit.

2. Distress Tolerance

What It Encompasses

Distress-tolerance skills help us survive intense emotion without making things worse (Linehan 2015).

They include grounding, safe distraction, self-soothing, and radical acceptance (Robins 2002)—the ability to say, *"This is my reality right now, even if I don't like it."*

How It Helps

When crises come, these skills keep us afloat until the storm passes (Neacsiu et al. 2010). They teach endurance, patience, and faith under pressure.

How It's Practiced

Distress tolerance is the art of staying present when everything in us wants to escape.

In DBT, it may involve simple actions—changing temperature, breathing deeply, or focusing on a single truth—to calm the body so the soul can breathe. Spiritually, it's learning to remain with God in the wilderness instead of running from it. It's whispering, *"I can't control this wave, but I can cling to You until it passes."*

Every act of staying becomes an act of faith.

Biblical Parallel

"In this world you will have trouble. But take heart! I have overcome the world" (John 16:33).

Faith and distress tolerance both teach perseverance—trusting that God's peace will return.

3. Emotion Regulation

What It Encompasses

Emotion-regulation skills teach us to understand, name, and influence emotions (Gratz and Roemer 2004).

They aim to reduce emotional vulnerability through caring for the body, increasing positive experiences, and practicing opposite action—doing the healthy thing even when we don't feel like it (Linehan 2015).

How It Helps

Emotions are messengers, not enemies. These skills help us listen to them without being controlled by them, replacing reactivity with stability.

How It's Practiced

Emotion regulation reminds us that feelings were never meant to be dictators—they are signals, not steering wheels. In DBT, this looks like caring for our physical needs, noticing patterns, and choosing responses aligned with truth rather than impulse.

Spiritually, it's learning to let the Holy Spirit be the compass of our hearts—guiding us back to center when emotion pulls us off course.

We practice discernment: noticing the wave, naming it, and choosing to ride it with wisdom instead of fear.

Biblical Parallel

"A gentle answer turns away wrath, but a harsh word stirs up anger" (Proverbs 15:1).

The Holy Spirit cultivates emotional wisdom—the grace to respond rather than react.

4. Interpersonal Effectiveness

What It Encompasses

This module focuses on relationships: expressing needs clearly, setting boundaries (Linehan 2015), saying no when necessary, and maintaining self-respect while caring for others.

How It Helps

It teaches balance—assertiveness with kindness. These skills improve communication, restore trust, and sustain healthy connections.

How It's Practiced

Interpersonal effectiveness is love with structure. It's learning to speak truth with gentleness, to listen with empathy, and to honor both our voice and the other's humanity.

DBT gives us language for this balance—how to assert needs without losing compassion (Fruzzetti 2007), how to set boundaries without building walls. Spiritually, it's what Jesus modeled: grace that never lies, truth that never wounds. Communication becomes healing when our words build bridges instead of barriers.

Biblical Parallel

"Speak the truth in love" (Ephesians 4:15).

DBT teaches what Jesus lived—communication rooted in both truth and grace.

How These Modules Work Together

Each module is part of a greater rhythm when integrated spiritually:

- Mindfulness helps us *notice* God's presence.

- Distress Tolerance helps us *trust* Him in the storm.

- Emotion Regulation helps us *yield* to His Spirit.

- Interpersonal Effectiveness helps us *reflect* His character in community.

Together, they nurture a life that is centered, resilient, and guided by wisdom (Linehan 2015)—what Scripture calls *"the mind of the Spirit"* (Romans 8:27 ESV).

Closing Thought

This overview isn't meant to replace therapy—it's meant to build understanding.

As you move forward, you'll see how DBT's practical wisdom and Scripture's eternal truth come together in the pages ahead—guiding us toward a life of emotional wholeness and spiritual peace.

Helpful Resources

For readers who wish to explore DBT directly from its clinical sources:

- Linehan, Marsha M. 2015. *DBT Skills Training Manual* (2nd ed.). The Guilford Press.

- Behavioral Tech—official DBT training site: www.behavioraltech.org

- Linehan Institute: https://linehaninstitute.org

- National Education Alliance for Borderline Personality Disorder (NEABPD): www.borderlinepersonalitydisorder.org

PART I

From the Divided Mind to the Renewed Integrated Mind

"The mind governed by the flesh is death, but the mind governed by the Spirit is life and peace."

—Romans 8:6

"Do not conform to the pattern of this world, but be transformed by the renewing of your mind."

—Romans 12:2

Every human being lives with a divided mind—pulled between emotion and reason, flesh and spirit. Dialectical Behavior Therapy (DBT) describes these tensions as *Emotion Mind* and *Reason Mind*, and invites us to find *Wise Mind*—the integrated space where truth and feeling meet. Based on Scripture (Romans 8:27), I will call this same idea "the Mind of the Spirit, " where divine wisdom and human experience are brought into alignment with God.

This part of the journey explores how DBT's skills like mindfulness and dialectical balance can become spiritual disciplines of awareness and surrender—practices that lead to the renewing of our minds in Christ. Here, evidence-based skills become instruments of grace, and spiritual formation becomes a process of integration: learning to think, feel, and live from the mind of the Spirit.

CHAPTER 1

Emotion Mind:
The Mind of the Flesh

The Morning After the Darkness

I still remember the taste of that morning—oatmeal, coffee, and fear.

It was March 2015, my first day returning to work after six months on disability. I had just been diagnosed with bipolar disorder. My first boyfriend since becoming a Christian—the one I trusted enough to tell—broke up with me over text when I shared my diagnosis. My psychiatrist was exploring different cocktails of medications that left me dizzy, sleepless, and hollow. I'd been laid off from a job I loved, creating youth-leadership programs for teens and young adults with trauma and schizophrenia. During those months, I sank into the couch and into despair, binge-watching *The Walking Dead* until I felt like a zombie myself.

When I finally accepted a temporary job at a real-estate firm—far from the purpose-filled career I'd hoped for—I thought I was starting over. But as I sat on my red couch that morning, oatmeal bowl in hand, I realized I was still just trying to survive.

My roommate slept, and her tiny chihuahua, "Coco," snored on the floor. Everything looked peaceful. But inside, it was war.

"You're disgusting."
"No man will ever want you."
"You used to be strong, now you're weak."
"God's disappointed in you."

The accusations came like waves until I could hardly breathe. My chest tightened, my legs buzzed with energy, my mind screamed RUN, though there was nowhere to go. I was sitting in safety, but my body and mind believed I was in danger. After all, wherever I could run, my mind would follow.

That's when I began to understand: I wasn't just battling a diagnosis. I was battling a divided mind.

One part—the Mind of the Flesh—was ruled by emotion without truth: shame, fear, and self-loathing disguised as repentance. Another—the voice of Worldly Wisdom— was ruled by logic without grace: perfectionism, control, and the illusion that if I could just understand myself, I could fix myself. And somewhere beneath both was a whisper I hadn't yet learned to trust—the Mind of the Spirit—quiet but steady, saying, "Breathe. You are still here. I have not given up on you."

At that time, I didn't know how to describe these three voices. I just knew my mind was constantly at war with itself. Yet even in that chaos, I kept reaching for my Bible. I couldn't always feel God in the words, but I knew I needed them like oxygen.

Every morning, I opened Scripture even when my heart felt numb, and my thoughts screamed louder than the gentle whispers of God's Word. Sometimes I read only a few verses before I broke down crying. Other times, I clung to one line—reading it over and over and struggling to believe it.

The Bible wasn't a comfort at first; it was an anchor. It didn't stop the storm, but it kept me from floating away.

During that same season, I also began doing Dialectical Behavioral Therapy (DBT) modules once a week. Eventually, I would complete all of them over the course of 18 months. DBT gave me practical tools to help me observe, name, and navigate the emotional chaos I lived in daily.

One skill stood out above the rest: the concept of Wise Mind[1]—the balanced place between Emotion

---

[1] Wise Mind is a core concept in Dialectical Behavior Therapy (DBT), repr[...] the balanced integration of emotion and reason. It is [...]he "inner wisdom" available when a person is simultane-[...]entered, and able to access both logic and emotion without [...]ed by either (Linehan 2015).

Mind[2] and Reason Mind, where both truth and feeling can coexist.

At first, I didn't realize it, but what DBT called Wise Mind mirrored what Scripture was teaching me about the Mind of the Spirit. Both invited me to pause between reaction and response, to breathe, to notice, and to let truth—not fear—be my guide. Both taught me that peace wasn't found in suppressing emotion or mastering logic, but in integrating them under something higher—what DBT called "wisdom," and what the Bible called "the Spirit of Truth."

Looking back, I can see that what I thought was me "barely hanging on" was actually the Spirit interceding through my daily practice of reading the Bible. Even when I couldn't pray, the Spirit was praying me back to life. Even when my mind was at war, the Spirit was gently teaching me to regulate not just my emotions, but my *awareness*—to locate myself somewhere deeper than fear or reason.

Romans 8:26–27 describes it perfectly:

At times we don't even know how to pray, or know the best things to ask for. But the Holy Spirit rises up within us to super-intercede on our behalf, pleading to God with emotional sighs too deep for words.

---

[2] Emotion Mind in DBT is the state where feelings are intense, overwhelming, and often interpreted as facts. It is marked by impulsivity, reactivity, and difficulty accessing logic or long-term perspective (Linehan 2015).

God, the searcher of the heart, knows fully our long-ings . . . because the Holy Spirit passionately pleads before God for us, His holy ones, in perfect harmony with God's plan and our destiny. (TPT)

In that season, I didn't have eloquent prayers or spiritual triumphs—more often, I just sobbed or felt numb. But I kept opening my Bible, kept attending DBT sessions, kept whispering, *"God, see me. God, help me."* And somehow, that was enough.

That daily act of showing up—to Scripture, to therapy, to stillness—became the doorway through which the Mind of the Spirit began to teach me how to hope again.

Looking back, I can see that DBT wasn't separate from God's work; it was one of His instruments. The Spirit used those weekly sessions like scaffolding around a fragile struc-ture—practical skills that created space for spiritual truth to lay a foundation. Therapy gave me awareness and the words to identify my emotions, but Scripture gave me the power to transform them. Together, therapy and Scripture became grace and truth in motion: skill and Spirit working side by side. The same God who inspired prophets and poets was also teaching me through DBT handouts and homework that spirituality isn't the absence of struggle; it's learning to stay present in it with God.

The Mind of the Flesh—Emotion Without Truth

States of the Mind
The Mind of the Spirit Integration

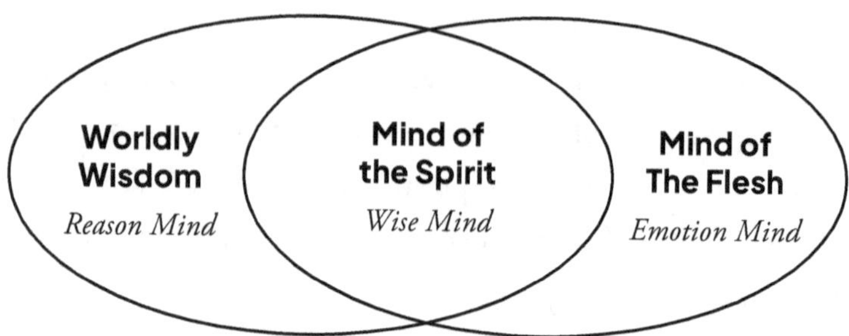

In Dialectical Behavioral Therapy (DBT) terms, this is Emotion Mind—the state where feelings turn into facts and every emotion demands obedience. Spiritually, Paul calls it *"the mind governed by the flesh,"* a mind that leads to death— not just physical death, but the slow dying of faith, hope, and love, the very things that keep us integrated, alive, and whole (Romans 8:6). Paul is not condemning emotion here; he is describing what happens when fear and self-protection lead the mind instead of the Spirit.

When I was in that state, I wasn't running from God— my true source of love—I was drowning in how I *felt* about Him. My thoughts became a storm of shame that sounded religious enough to believe.

Emotion Mind told me:

You are too broken to be used by God.
You aren't doing "well" spiritually.

Your diagnosis is God putting limits on how He plans
to use you.
Your emotions prove you lack conviction.

And I believed it.

That's what DBT helped me name. In therapy, I was learning that Emotion Mind is real—it's powerful, overwhelming, and convincing—but it's not the full truth. Emotion Mind interprets pain as danger and feelings as facts. DBT gave me language for what Scripture had already revealed: that when emotions lead without truth, they become tyrants.

Emotion Mind without grace clings to comfort and control. It confuses counterfeit comforts for survival and numbing for rest. So I reached for false peace—binging Netflix, eating junk food, isolating. I thought I was recovering, but I was retreating. I thought I was protecting my faith, but I was silencing my heart.

The Mind of the Flesh doesn't only crave pleasure; it craves escape. It's where pain becomes identity and emotion becomes authority. Emotion itself is not sin; it is part of being human. The danger begins when emotion becomes disconnected from truth, presence, and communion with God.

That's the tragedy of the flesh: operating from our emotions is disguised as self-protection, using emotion as a barrier that blocks the very healing and rescue from God we're desperate for.

Then mercy found me.

Lamentations says, "The steadfast love of the Lord never ceases; His mercies never come to an end; they are new every morning . . ." (3:22–23 ESV).

Each morning I woke up was proof that God's mercy hadn't given up on me, even when I felt filled with shame and guilt for my actions or inaction from the day before. Each sunrise was another invitation to start again.

That realization shifted everything. I didn't need to fight my emotions; I needed to invite God into them.

Around the same time, DBT was teaching me to *observe* and *name* my feelings without judgment, to breathe before reacting, to find the small space between impulse and action.[3] I began to see that this pause—the moment of awareness before reaction—was holy ground.

That's where I started to sense the presence of what DBT called Wise Mind—the quiet, centered awareness that holds both emotion and reason together.

Wise Mind reminded me of the Mind of the Spirit Paul describes.
Both are still, discerning, and compassionate.
Both whisper truth into chaos and help us choose life over reaction.
Both make space for grace.

---

[3] DBT encourages developing awareness of the space between stimulus and response—a mindfulness-based intervention that increases emotional regulation and reduces impulsivity (Linehan 2015; Bishop et al. 2004).

When I practiced DBT, I was learning emotional regulation; when I prayed and opened Scripture, I was experiencing spiritual transformation. And slowly, the two began to overlap.

DBT showed me *how* to pause. The Spirit showed me *who* was in the pause.

That morning on the couch became the beginning of surrender—the first moment I stopped letting emotion rule me and started letting the Spirit teach me.

The Bible says the flesh is a gravitational pull that drags our minds toward self-protection and self-gratification: "Those who are motivated by the flesh only pursue what benefits themselves . . . but the mind-set controlled by the Spirit finds life and peace" (Romans 8:5-6 TPT).

That morning, my emotions became my gods. Fear demanded obedience. Shame issued verdicts. Anxiety sentenced me to isolation.

When we live from the Mind of the Flesh, emotions act like false prophets. They shout, "Comfort yourself!" promising relief but delivering ruin. God is whispering, "Let Me in—I will comfort you."

The Bible reminds us, "So now the case is closed. There remains no accusing voice of condemnation against those who are joined in life-union with Jesus . . ." (Romans 8:1 TPT).

The Mind of the Flesh doesn't know that verdict. It keeps reopening a trial God already dismissed. It rehearses guilt. It confuses conviction with condemnation and repentance with self-punishment.

Only when I began to believe that *the case was closed* did mercy start re-wiring my emotions.

The Spirit wasn't asking me to suppress my feelings—He was teaching me to submit them to Him.

And that submission wasn't silence; it was surrender.

Pause and Practice

1. Notice your storm. Take a slow breath and ask yourself: *What emotion is trying to take over right now?* Name it honestly without judging it. (DBT calls this "observing" and "describing."[4])

2. Invite truth into it. Say—*The case is closed. There is no condemnation for those who are in Christ Jesus* (Romans 8:1). Let that truth speak louder than your feelings.

3. Find the holy pause. Before reacting or reaching for comfort, pause for just five seconds. Breathe. This small space is where the Spirit waits to meet you—your first glimpse of Wise Mind, or what Scripture calls the *Mind of the Spirit.*

---

[4] "Observe" and "Describe" are part of DBT's Mindfulness skills, designed to help individuals notice internal experiences without judgment and label them accurately. These foundational skills help break automatic emotional reactions (Linehan 2015).

4. Surrender, not suppression.[5] Tell God what you feel, and then release control of it. You don't have to fix it; you just have to invite Him into it.

5. Affirm this truth: "I am safe to feel because I am loved. I am free to surrender because the case is closed."

When We Try to Light Our Own Fires

Stillness became the hinge between death and life. For the first time, I stopped trying to "light my own fires." Isaiah 50 became my mirror, ". . . Are any of you groping in the dark without light? Trust in the faithful name of Yahweh and rely on your God. But if you presume to light your own torch, you are playing with fire . . . it will take you down into torment!" (v. 10-11 TPT).

That verse named exactly what both my emotion and my intellect had been doing—creating their own rescue plans.

Emotion Mind or the Mind of the Flesh built its fire from panic: *Run. Numb. Protect yourself.* Reason Mind or Worldly Wisdom built its fire from pride: *Analyze. Fix. Perform.*

But both flames consumed me.

In DBT, we talk about how Emotion Mind and Reason

---

[5] Radical Acceptance is a DBT technique involving complete openness to the present moment, acknowledging reality without resistance. It is not agreement, but a skill to reduce suffering caused by fighting what is beyond control (Linehan 2015).

Mind each hold partial truths, but neither can see the whole picture. When they operate separately, they burn us—one in chaos, the other in control. But there's a third space called Wise Mind—a quiet center that holds both logic and emotion, awareness and acceptance, truth and tenderness.

Spiritually, I began to see that Wise Mind was not something I had to *achieve*; it was Someone I had to *listen to and invite in*. What DBT called Wise Mind, Scripture called the Mind of the Spirit.[6]

Both invite us to stop lighting fires of our own understanding and wait for the true light of God's presence.

It was that waiting, bearing up under the burden of the pain[7] discomfort, fear, and the unknown that was the hardest discipline of all.

My Fires of Self-Rescue

This is how sin often begins—not with rebellion, but with disconnection: the moment we try to survive without God's

---

[6] DBT's Wise Mind is often described as a non-religious form of inner intuition or centered awareness. Its function parallels spiritual traditions that emphasize discernment, stillness, and grounded presence (Linehan 2015; Kristeller 2003).

[7] Distress Tolerance skills in DBT teach individuals how to endure emotional pain without engaging in harmful behaviors, focusing on acceptance, non-judgment, and survival strategies during crisis moments (Linehan 2015).

presence. Stillness has never come naturally to me. When I'm triggered by something that stirs up old trauma or makes me feel anxious and unsafe, my first instinct is to run—not physically, but through motion. I light my own fires. I fill my days with projects, responsibilities, and goals that look purposeful on the outside but are often panic in disguise.[8]

When I feel pain rising, I chase distraction: another project, another ambition, another plan to prove I'm okay. I've buried myself in endless work, climbed professional ladders, and sought affirmation from people—anything to feel like I'm escaping the ache inside. For a while, it works. The adrenaline of achievement feels like progress. The attention feels like comfort. But underneath, my soul is still restless, my body exhausted, and my spirit disconnected.

I've learned that this kind of striving is just another form of self-rescue. It's the Mind of the Flesh disguised as productivity. My anxiety dresses up as ambition, and my fear of being powerless pretends to be passion. But every time I try to rescue myself, I end up ignoring the very places in me that need God most—my heart, my health, my emotions, my relationships.

Those seasons of overdrive have taught me that success cannot heal wounds that only surrender can. The more

---

[8] In DBT, Emotion Mind often leads to ineffective attempts to escape pain through impulsive or avoidant behaviors—sometimes called "short-term relief, long-term suffering." This aligns with the metaphor of pursuing "false fires" that destabilize rather than soothe (Linehan 2015).

I light my own fires, the more I burn myself out. What I really need is not another plan, but presence—the presence of God that meets me in stillness, not in striving.

When I finally stop running, I realize how much I've been prolonging my pain by avoiding it. The healing I need is never found in achievement; it's found in awareness—the quiet recognition of where I've tried to save myself, so I can surrender those places back to the One who actually saves. Every time I choose stillness over striving, I find that God's light burns steadier than any fire I could build.

Psalm 62 gives language to this:

I am standing in absolute stillness, silent before the One I love, waiting as long as it takes for Him to rescue me. Only God is my Savior, and He will not fail me . . . For He alone is my safe place . . . Trust only in God every moment! Tell Him all your troubles and pour out your heart-longings to Him . . . Pause in His presence. (v. 5–8 TPT)

This passage taught me that stillness isn't passivity—it's a protest against self-reliance.

It's choosing to let the match fall from your hand. It's believing that the darkness isn't punishment, but preparation for divine light to come rushing in. As the prophet Micah says, "Though I have fallen, I will rise. Though I sit in darkness, the Lord will be my light.

He will bring me out into the light; I will see His right-eousness" (7:8-9).

Micah didn't deny the darkness. He sat in it, trusting that God Himself would plead his case.

The Mind of the Flesh says, *I must escape the dark.*
Worldly Wisdom says, *I must understand the dark.*
The Mind of the Spirit says, *I will sit in the dark until God becomes my light.*

That realization began to free me from the addiction of self-rescue. It also helped me understand what DBT had been training me for all along—how to tolerate distress without immediately fixing or fleeing. In DBT terms, this was *distress tolerance*; in spiritual terms, it was *trust*.

Learning to stay still, to breathe through discomfort without numbing or analyzing it, became my practice of faith. Every time I chose to wait in the dark with God instead of lighting my own fire, I was building the muscle of learning to let the Mind of the Spirit lead—the inner space where my humanity and His divinity could finally meet and walk together.

Later, when I read 1 Kings 19, Elijah's exhaustion felt like my own. He had outrun prophets and miracles, yet collapsed under a broom tree and begged to die. God didn't scold him or demand performance; He sent food, rest, and finally—a whisper. The verse says, ". . . after the fire came a gentle whisper . . . When Elijah heard it, he pulled his cloak over his face . . ." (v.12–13).

That whisper is the Mind of the Spirit—truth wrapped in tenderness, strength that does not shout, peace that enters the room without demanding perfection.

And sometimes wisdom is knowing the Spirit isn't found in the fire we build to survive, but in the quiet after it burns out.

Pause and Practice—Letting the Fire Go Out

1. Observe.
    Pause for ten seconds.
    Notice what's happening inside you—your breath, your body, your urge to fix, flee, or perform.
    Simply observe without judging it. This is the first step toward peace.

2. Describe.
    Name your "fire."
    What are you reaching for when you feel unsafe—control, work, comfort, or distraction?
    Whisper it honestly to God. Naming breaks its power.

3. Participate.
    Take one mindful breath with the Spirit.
    Inhale: *"Lord, You are my light."*
    Exhale: *"I release the fire I built."*

This is where emotion and truth meet—the Mind of the Spirit guiding your next step.

4. Radical Acceptance.
    Read Psalm 62:5 (TPT)—
    "I am standing in absolute stillness, silent before the One I love . . ."
    Accept the moment as it is. You don't have to fix it; you only have to stay with God in it.

5. Realign.
    Whisper a reminder from Romans 8:1: *The case is closed.*
    Let grace quiet the guilt.
    Then journal one sentence:

Affirmation:

Every time I choose stillness over striving, I am choosing trust over torment.

The Lord Himself is my light.

Emotion isn't the only counterfeit light; sometimes reason builds its own fire. In the next chapter, we'll look at how logic without love—Worldly Wisdom—can keep us just as far from the warmth of God's presence, and how reason without grace can harden the heart that God longs to heal.

CHAPTER 2

Reason Mind:
The Wisdom of the World

The Fortress of Logic

There's another part of the mind that feels safer than raw emotion. It dresses itself in reason, professionalism, and even theology. Reason itself is a gift from God; it becomes Worldly Wisdom only when it is used to replace dependence on Him rather than deepen relationship with Him. It says, *If I can understand it, I can control it.* That's what Scripture calls Worldly Wisdom—and what DBT calls Reason Mind.[9]

---

[9] Reason Mind in DBT refers to a state of thinking grounded primarily in logic, facts, and analysis. It is helpful for planning and problem-solving but becomes ineffective when it overrides emotional awareness or interpersonal connection (Linehan 2015).

It isn't loud like Emotion Mind; it's efficient. It organizes, intellectualizes, and polishes pain until it looks respectable. It builds charts where chaos once lived and labels where feelings once roared. Reason Mind can look holy, disciplined, or even wise—but without grace, it becomes a fortress containing the chaos inside instead of a sanctuary within. 1 Corinthians says, "Knowledge puffs up, but love builds up. Those who think they know something do not yet know as they ought. But whoever loves God is known by God" (8:1-3).

Reason Mind and Worldly Wisdom both share a single obsession: control instead of closeness. They believe that clarity equals safety—that if we can explain the pain, we can escape it. But understanding is not the same as a relationship that leads to transformation.

Spiritual Performance and the Illusion of Control

Even Jesus warned that spiritual activity without intimacy is empty:

> Not everyone who says to Me, 'Lord, Lord,' will enter the kingdom of heaven, but only the one who does the will of My Father . . . Many will say to me on that day, 'Lord, Lord, did we not prophesy in your name, and in your name drive out demons and in your name perform many miracles?' Then I will tell them plainly, 'I never knew you . . . ' (Matthew 7:21–23)

I realized that even "doing everything right" in faith could become another form of Worldly Wisdom. It hides behind good behavior and spiritual credentials. It convinces us that precision, polish, and theological fluency equal holiness. This is how sin often disguises itself—not as rebellion, but as self-sufficiency lived apart from God's presence. But Jesus came to redeem what was lost, to reconcile the broken to Himself, so He would be known, we would be fully known by Him, and participate fully in His Kingdom.

Clinical–Spiritual Bridge

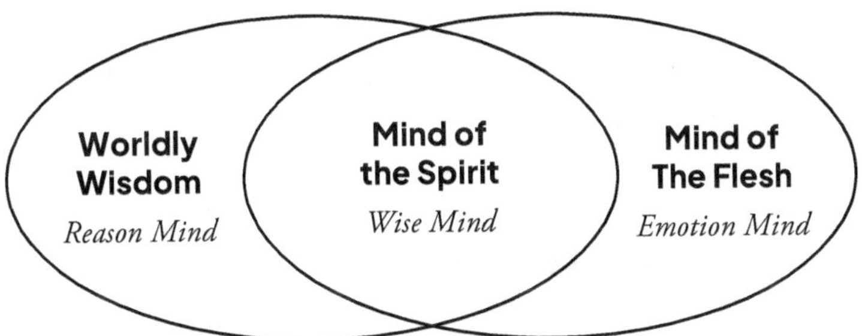

In DBT, Reason Mind is useful when we need order and logic, but it becomes dangerous when it crowds out empathy and closeness. Spiritually, Worldly Wisdom does the same thing: it values knowing *about* God over *being known* by Him. It values earning God's favor over intimacy with Jesus. To receive the gift of grace, His unmerited favor where and when we need it most, we must be in relationship with Him.

When I lived from that part of my mind—performing stability—I quoted Scripture and pretended to manage my moods, but I couldn't feel God, His love, His healing, or His hope. My logic was precise, but my heart was cold, hard, and unbelieving. I was living in what DBT would call *over-controlled behavior*:[10] externally composed, internally disconnected, despairing, and enslaved to fear.

I could analyze my triggers, recite my verses, and still miss the whisper of the Spirit that wanted communion and compassion more than comprehension.

Worldly Wisdom says, *You are saved by understanding and doing.*

The Mind of the Spirit says, *You are saved by being known by God.*

From Dissection to Discernment

Romans 8:2 says, "the law of the Spirit of life in Christ Jesus has set you free from the law of sin and death." That

---

[10] Overcontrol describes patterns of emotional inhibition, perfectionism, excessive self-control, and difficulty expressing vulnerability—traits associated with chronic distress and relational disconnection. DBT-RO (Radically Open DBT) identifies this as a core driver of psychological rigidity (Lynch 2018).

means even our intellect—our need to reason everything through—can be reconciled to God. The Spirit doesn't discard logic; He purifies it. He takes our analytical precision and turns it into discernment. He turns information into intimacy.

In DBT, the bridge between Emotion Mind and Reason Mind is Wise Mind[11]—the integrated awareness where truth and feeling collaborate instead of competing. That's the same place the Spirit lives. Wise Mind listens for the *gentle whisper* Elijah heard, the quiet faith that transcends intellectual proof.

When I began to notice this overlap, my therapy sessions and my prayer life started to merge.

The Spirit would meet me in my DBT worksheets as surely as in Scripture—teaching me that mindfulness was just another way of saying, *"Be still and know that I am God"* (Psalm 46:10).

Observing without judgment became repentance without shame.

Describing my inner world became my confession.

Participating fully in the present moment became standing in awe of God.

---

[11] Wise Mind is the integrated state where Emotion Mind and Reason Mind work together, allowing the individual to access inner wisdom, clarity, and balanced judgment (Linehan 2015).

Slowly, I realized that God was not asking me to stop thinking—He was asking me to think *with* Him. Worldly Wisdom has taught me to dissect. The Spirit was teaching me to discern. DBT had taught me to notice. The Spirit was teaching me to *listen.*

And that's the transformation:

Logic is no longer my light, but my lamp—faithful, limited, and surrendered to a greater flame.

Pause and Practice

1. Name your Reason Mind patterns. Where do you seek control through analysis, rules, or spiritual performance?

2. Integrate, don't eliminate. Invite the Spirit to sit beside your logic. Ask, *"What truth am I missing because I'm trying to manage instead of trusting?"*

3. Integrate DBT + Prayer:[12]

    - *Observe* → Notice your thoughts without judgment.

    - *Describe* → Speak them honestly to God.

------

[12] "Observe," "Describe," and "Participate" are DBT's core Mindfulness "What Skills," designed to build non-judgmental awareness and help individuals shift from reactive processing to grounded presence (Linehan 2015).

- *Participate* → Let His presence, not your performance, lead the moment.

4. Whisper Romans 8:6: *"The mind controlled by the
   Spirit finds life and peace."*

When Control Pretends to Be Faith

I see now how often I've lived from the fortress of Worldly
Wisdom without realizing it.

Control has never felt like rebellion to me—it's felt like
responsibility, like love, like faith in motion. But when I
trace the root of it, I find fear.[13]

There are moments when I try to earn outcomes through
effort, especially in the areas that matter most to me—our
foster sons, my marriage, my ministry, my work. I tell myself
that if I can advocate clearly enough, pray faithfully enough,
perform graciously enough, maybe everything will turn out
right. I've treated faith like a formula, and peace like a prize
for performance. But God's will has never been something
to master or manage; it is something to abide in. That's not
communion; that's control in religious clothing.

Other times, I hide behind competence and overachieve-
ment when I'm anxious or afraid. I fill my life with projects,

---

[13] DBT research shows that both overcontrol and emotional avoidance
are often rooted in fear—fear of rejection, uncertainty, or loss of identity—which can drive rigid thinking or excessive problem-solving efforts
(Lynch 2018; Linehan 2015).

goals, and endless productivity, mistaking motion for meaning. When I can't feel God's presence, I analyze Him. When I'm afraid to be misunderstood, I overexplain. When I feel helpless, I over function. And though these habits make me look strong, they quietly starve the part of me that needs tenderness, rest, and trust.

Even my deepest acts of love can drift into control if I'm not careful. I've tried to fix what only the Spirit can heal— systems, relationships, outcomes, people. I've mistaken being faithful with being in charge. But God keeps showing me that control and communion cannot coexist. One requires striving; the other requires surrendered trust.

I'm learning that intimacy with God doesn't grow through mastery but through mutuality. It's less about doing things *for* Him and more about being *with* Him. He doesn't need my flawless execution; He desires my honest presence. When I stop managing and start abiding, I feel His whisper again: "I don't need your perfection. I want your participation."

The longer I walk with Jesus, the more I realize that my logic was never meant to lead me—it was meant to kneel beside my love. I don't have to understand to be held. I don't have to earn peace to receive it. I don't have to prove my faith to be known by the One who gave it to me.

Control builds a fortress; communion builds a home. And I want to live where He dwells.

The Turning Point: From Control to Communion

I wish I could say I've mastered this—living fully from the Mind of the Spirit, abiding instead of analyzing—but the truth is, it's very hard for me. I bend toward my Emotion Mind, but when I'm afraid of being misunderstood or rejected, I swing to Reason Mind—polished, composed, appearing "in control." It's not just about logic; it's about wanting to be acceptable—to God, to people, maybe even to myself.

I know what the Bible says. I know that grace isn't earned. But many days, I catch myself performing, as if stability and spiritual fluency will prove I belong. It's easier to talk about God than to talk to Him. Easier to interpret Scripture than to let Scripture interpret me. Easier to look "faithful" than to be fully seen.

That's when the Spirit gently whispers a word that undoes me every time: "Abide."

Abide in Me, and I in you. As the branch cannot bear fruit by itself unless it abides in the vine, neither can you unless you abide in Me. I am the vine; you are the branches. Whoever abides in Me and I in him bears much fruit, for apart from Me you can do nothing. (John 15:4–5)

That word isn't a command to perform; it's an invitation to stay. Abiding isn't about understanding—it's about union.[14] It's the opposite of control. It's learning to *remain* in love even when I can't prove my worth or make sense of my emotions.

In DBT, this mirrors the move from Reason Mind to Wise Mind—the place where logic surrenders to awareness, and awareness surrenders to truth. I know the skills: observe, describe, participate, and regulate. I know how to pause, breathe, and find that inner stillness.

But even knowing doesn't make it easy.

Sometimes I find myself studying Scripture like a map,[15] looking for a formula instead of a Father.

Other times, I freeze in fear—afraid that my emotions disqualify me from being "spiritual enough."

That's when I have to remember what the Bible says in Romans 8:9-11, "When the Spirit of Christ empowers your life, you are not dominated by the flesh but by the Spirit . . . His life-giving Spirit imparts life to you because you are fully accepted by God."

That word—accepted—keeps saving me. Because even when I drift into self-reliance or over-control, the Spirit keeps drawing me back to God's presence. He reminds me

---

[14] Radical Acceptance in DBT parallels spiritual practices of surrender and abiding, emphasizing full openness to reality without resistance or attempts to force control (Linehan 2015; Hayes et al. 1999).

[15] Excessive analysis and rumination are cognitive processes linked to Reason Mind dominance and overcontrol. DBT aims to shift individuals from rumination toward experiential awareness (Lynch 2018).

that understanding will never make me righteous—only rela-tionship will.

And honestly? I'm still learning how to live that way. I still slide into performing when I feel unsafe, or retreat into logic when life feels too painful to feel. But each time I notice it, I get another chance to practice Wise Mind[16]—not as a skill, but as a surrender.

To pause.
To breathe.
To remember, "Abide."

This is what integration looks like for me—not perfection, but participation. Not mastering faith, but meeting God in my weakness. It's the long practice of letting my intellect kneel beside my emotions at the feet of grace.

That's where the Mind of the Spirit meets me—not when I finally "get it," but when I finally stop pretending I do.

Pause and Practice

1. Notice your default. When life feels uncertain, do you move toward Emotion Mind (react) or Reason Mind (control)?

---

[16] Returning to Wise Mind is a central mindfulness strategy in DBT—a repeated re-centering practice rather than a permanent state (Linehan 2015).

2. Name the fear. What are you afraid would happen if you simply abided instead of analyzing or performing?

3. Return to presence. Whisper John 15:4, *"Abide in Me, and I in you."*

4. Integrate DBT + Faith:

   - *Observe* → "I see my need to control."

   - *Describe* → "I'm afraid of not being enough."

   - *Participate* → "Spirit, meet me in this moment."

When intellect finally kneels beside emotion, something holy awakens between them.

The Mind of the Spirit—the quiet integration of wisdom and love, and reason and reverence, is unlocked.

In the next chapter, we'll explore what it means to live from that space where mindfulness becomes God-fullness, and peace begins to guard the heart and mind in Christ.

CHAPTER 3

The Mind of the Spirit— The Path to Integration

There are moments—fleeting, holy, and often unexpected—when everything quiets.

Not because the storm has stopped, but because something greater is present within it.

That's what I've come to recognize as the Mind of the Spirit—what DBT calls Wise Mind.[17]

---

[17] Wise Mind is the integrated state in DBT where emotion and reason are held together, allowing a person to act from a place of balanced awareness, intuition, and clarity (Linehan 2015).

States of the Mind
The Mind of the Spirit Integration

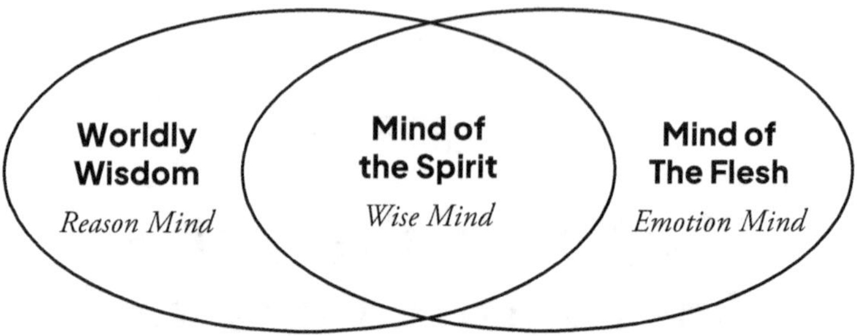

The Mind of the Spirit unites what the flesh and the world tear apart.[18] It holds both truth and emotion, both intellect and empathy. It's where grace and grounding meet.

The Spirit validates emotion without indulging it, honors logic without idolizing it. It's the inner regulator that lets us tell the truth about pain while remaining faithful to hope. It allows us to feel deeply without being consumed and to think clearly without growing cold.

The Mind of the Spirit, as we learn to sit in discomfort and wait on God, helps us create space—a holy gap between a trigger and a reaction.[19] That gap is where we find God:

---

[18] DBT describes Wise Mind as the convergence of Emotion Mind (emotion-driven, reactive state) and Reason Mind (logic-driven, analytical state), forming a third state where both systems work in harmony (Linehan 2015).

[19] DBT emphasizes mindfulness practices that increase one's ability to observe internal experiences and insert a pause between stimulus and

guiding us, grounding us, and helping us learn to respond to life in alignment with our biblical values, in step with the Holy Spirit, and in harmony with God's will. That will is not a guarantee that circumstances will go the way we want—it is the invitation to remain in communion with Him and respond from His presence, even when life is not yet healed. It's in that small but holy pause that reactivity becomes reflection, and reflection becomes awe of God. God's will is what love looks like in real time. The Kingdom of God doesn't always change the external storm immediately, but it does begin changing who is ruling inside me. That is where integration starts.

When I was fourteen, I learned what it meant to live from that space for the first time. It was the season of my most radical transformation—not because I was strong, but because I was starving, and I learned to feed on Scripture.

The Word of God became my bread.

> I am the bread of life. Your ancestors ate the manna in the wilderness, yet they died. But here is the bread that comes down from heaven, which anyone may eat and not die. I am the living bread that came down from heaven. Whoever eats this bread will live forever. (John 6:48–51)

---

response—reducing impulsive or automatic reactions (Bishop et al. 2004; Linehan 2015).

At fourteen, I consumed Scripture like my abuelita's tortillas; it was my comfort food. It was the one thing that steadied me when everything else felt unstable. I didn't yet know words like *Wise Mind* or *emotional regulation*—I just knew that every time I opened the Bible, peace entered the room.

John begins his gospel by identifying Jesus as the Word made flesh: "In the beginning was the Word, and the Word was with God, and the Word was God" (John 1:1).

When Jesus later told His followers to "eat His flesh" and "drink His blood," many were offended. But I think what He meant was this: *consume My life, My Word, My way. Take My example into your body, your thoughts, your choices. Let My truth be what nourishes you and regulates your responses.*

That's what the Mind of the Spirit teaches us—to respond in ways that align with His will, not our wounds. To digest His Word until it becomes part of our emotional and spiritual metabolism and to embody God's Kingdom. In this book, I mean God's Kingdom the way Jesus taught it: the active reign of God—where truth, love, justice, and peace begin ruling first in us, then through us.

Today, I still make it my goal to consume the Bread of Life daily to commune with God and embody His Kingdom—but it's harder than it used to be. My life at thirty-seven is more complex than it was at fourteen. I'm constantly racing—from meeting to meeting, project to project, responsibility to responsibility. Even when I finally sit down, my mind keeps running.

Adulting, managing mental health, and living in the physical world often leave little room for the Spirit to whisper from the spiritual one. There are days when I open my Bible and can't feel anything—just static in my brain and a dozen to-do lists tugging at my focus. I'll start a prayer and suddenly remember an email I forgot to send, groceries I need to order, or I receive a social media notification. My mind races for control, while my spirit whispers, *"Stay."* Those are the moments I practice noticing my racing thoughts, naming them in prayer, and breathing until I can sense His nearness again. Sometimes my body is still in survival mode even when my spirit is turning toward God—and that doesn't mean I'm failing; it means I'm healing. In those moments, I've often had to become creative in how I feed my soul.

I listen to Scripture songs during my commute. I use Bible apps that read the Word aloud while I walk, work, or wind down for bed. Sometimes I fall asleep with verses playing softly through my AirPods. Other times, I draw or journal Scriptures—turning the verses into images and prayers, so my hands can help my heart listen.

Each of these practices slows my thoughts and tunes my awareness to the Spirit. They help me hear Him speak just a little louder than my already verbose thoughts and demanding emotions.

They help me remember that the Word is not just something to read—it's Someone to receive.

My circumstances do not need to change to experience

peace, but my relationship with the Spirit does need to change. This is true whether I am starting a new temporary job, learning to manage medication, or facing uncertainty about my future. Inside, the storm begins to still when I embrace and draw near to the Mind of the Spirit.

The same God who met Elijah in a whisper was meeting me on that red couch in 2015.

That whisper became the rhythm of my healing:[20] love building where knowledge once puffed up, mercy replacing self-judgment, and peace surpassing understanding.

Paul describes this kind of peace in Philippians 4:6-7, "Do not be anxious about anything, but in every situation, by prayer and petition, with thanksgiving, present your requests to God. And the peace of God, which transcends all understanding, will guard your hearts and your minds in Christ Jesus."

That word *guard* stands out to me. The Spirit wasn't just comforting me; He was *protecting* me—from my own extremes, from the false fires I once lit. The Mind of the Spirit became my inner regulator[21]—the holy balance where

---

[20] Mindfulness practices in DBT regulate emotional intensity by grounding individuals in the present moment and reducing cognitive fusion with distressing emotions or thoughts (Linehan 2015; Hayes et al. 2011).

[21] Mindfulness-based practices support neural integration between emotional and cognitive brain regions, increasing coherence and resilience (Siegel 2012).

my emotions could cry, my intellect could question, and both could stay rooted in love.

DBT had given me the framework for Wise Mind; the Spirit filled it with life.

Wise Mind taught me mindfulness; the Spirit taught me *God-fullness.*[22] Wise Mind helped me observe; the Spirit helped me *abide.*

And together, they began rebuilding what years of fragmentation had broken—slowly, gently, faithfully.

I don't live here all the time. I still lose balance, swinging between reactivity and rigidity. But every time I return to stillness,[23] I find Him already waiting there—patient and unhurried, whispering, *"Be still. I'm here, you are safe with Me."*

That's the Mind of the Spirit. It's not a formula to master, but a friendship to cultivate. The Spirit isn't teaching me how to control life; He's teaching me how to stay with God inside it. It's not about control or knowing, but communion and trust.

Jesus lived from this place perfectly. He is the ultimate case study of the Mind of the Spirit in motion—feeling deeply, thinking clearly, obeying completely. His emotional

---

[22] Observe, Describe, and Participate are DBT's foundational Mindfulness "What Skills," designed to cultivate non-judgmental awareness and embodied presence (Linehan 2015).

[23] DBT's "How Skills"—Non-judgmentally, One-Mindfully, and Effectively—describe the manner in which mindfulness is practiced, enabling sustained emotional regulation and clarity (Linehan 2015).

life was not a weakness; it was worship. His wisdom was not about being right; it was about being *with* the Father.

In a future chapter, we'll look closely at how Jesus embodied this divine integration—how His peace came not from balance but from belonging, how His wisdom flowed not from control but from communion.

For now, I am still learning to listen for that same whisper that found me on the red couch years ago—to let the Spirit, not my emotions or intellect, write the final word.

And maybe that's the point of healing: not to live without storms, but to know who quiets them.

I still forget this truth daily. Some mornings I wake up in the Mind of the Flesh, anxious and striving; by afternoon, I'm buried in the Mind of the World, analyzing everything. But each time I pause long enough to breathe, the Spirit reminds me that integration isn't something I achieve—it's Someone I return to.[24] Every moment of awareness becomes an altar where peace meets me again.

Pause and Practice

1. Notice your gap. Where do you feel the space between a trigger and your reaction? Breathe into that gap—it's sacred ground. Invite God into it.

____

[24] In DBT, Wise Mind is not a static achievement but a practice of continually returning to a grounded, centered awareness amid emotional swings (Linehan 2015).

2. Nourish your spirit. Find one creative way to "consume the Bread of Life" today—listen to Scripture, sing it, draw it, or pray it out loud.

3. Align, don't analyze. When you're unsure how to respond, ask: *Does this align with my biblical values and the Spirit's peace?*

4. Whisper Philippians 4:7: *"And the peace of God, which transcends all understanding, will guard [my heart] and [my mind] in Christ Jesus."*

5. Rest: The goal isn't perfect stillness—it's a steady return to the One who meets you there.

PART II

The Practice:
Living from the Mind of
the Spirit

"Since we live by the Spirit, let us keep in step with the Spirit."

—Galatians 5:25

"Whatever you have learned or received or heard from me, or seen in me—put it into practice. And the God of peace will be with you."

—Philippians 4:9

If Part I revealed the divided mind and invited us toward integration, Part II calls us to live from that integration daily. This is where the Mind of the Spirit becomes a lived practice—a rhythm of awareness, truth, and grace embodied in our relationships, emotions, and choices.

Here, the skills of Dialectical Behavior Therapy (DBT)—mindfulness, distress tolerance, emotion regulation, and interpersonal effectiveness—become spiritual disciplines that train us to walk in step with the Spirit. The goal is not perfection but participation: to live with increasing alignment between what we believe, what we feel, and how we love. This is the practice of living from the Mind of the Spirit— moment by moment, breath by breath, as evidence-based skills become sacred habits that form us in Christ.

CHAPTER 4

Distress Tolerance: Sitting with God in the Wilderness

There are seasons when God does not remove the suffering, change the circumstances, or answer the prayer the way we asked. Chapter 4 explores what it means to remain with God in those moments—when faithfulness looks less like action and more like endurance.

What Is Distress Tolerance?

In DBT, *Distress Tolerance*[25] is the set of skills that help us survive emotional pain without making the moment worse.

---

[25] Distress Tolerance in DBT refers to crisis survival strategies designed to help individuals endure emotional pain without engaging in impulsive or destructive behaviors (Linehan 2015).

It's the ability to sit with reality when we cannot change it,[26] to withstand discomfort without collapsing into avoidance, impulsivity, or despair. Distress Tolerance doesn't remove suffering; it strengthens us to endure it skillfully, with clarity instead of chaos.

Spiritually, Distress Tolerance is the wilderness space[27]— the holy ground where we learn to breathe with God when nothing around us feels certain. It's where faith becomes more than belief; it becomes endurance, surrender, and deep internal resilience. It is the invitation to stay present with God in the places we most want to escape.

The Wilderness as Holy Ground

When I think back to that season of waiting for the court's decision about two of our foster sons—children my husband and I deeply loved and hoped to adopt—the memories feel suspended in time. Every day held its own ache: the kind that can't be prayed away, only lived through.

I remember sitting in silence after another tense hearing when the judge decided to extend the case another six

---

[26] Distress Tolerance emphasizes accepting the present moment as it is, focusing on endurance rather than emotional avoidance or suppression (Linehan 2015).

[27] Mindfulness-based therapies conceptualize emotional "wilderness" experiences as opportunities for cultivating resilience and tolerance for distress (Bishop et al. 2004).

months. I felt numb—mind racing through every possible outcome, yet there were no answers, only more waiting.

I was overwhelmed: early mornings, bedtime routines, court paperwork, therapy meetings, a full-time job, comforting toddlers acting out their trauma, and trying to stay attuned to my husband rather than reacting to him. I was emotionally and physically drained, living on empty. My prayers had become wordless—groans, really. They were somewhere between pleading and surrender. I wasn't just asking God to change the outcome, I was asking Him to keep me from breaking under the weight of the waiting.

At the time, I thought the wilderness meant I had done something wrong. Other people seemed to build their families easily; why did mine have to be so complicated, so costly? Maybe God had led me here to expose my weakness—to show me I wasn't strong enough to be a mom, let alone a foster-adoptive mom.

But slowly, Scripture began whispering a different story:

Jesus entered the wilderness *before* His ministry began.
David fled into caves *before* he ever wore a crown.
Moses wandered *before* he was called to lead.
Israel circled the desert *before* stepping into promise.

The wilderness is not where God abandons us—it's where He prepares us.

This Wilderness Season Is Preparation for Something Greater

There are days when I still feel isolated, exhausted, and completely drained. I wonder why God allows certain seasons to stretch on so long. I'm learning that God allowing is not the same as approving—and Scripture never portrays God as the author of harm, even when He allows human freedom and broken systems to run their course. And I've learned that God uses these wilderness seasons as a precursor *before* the promise.

Jesus went into the wilderness before beginning His ministry (Matthew 4:1–11). Paul spent years in the desert before becoming the great apostle (Galatians 1:15–18*)*. Israel had to go through the wilderness before entering the Promised Land (Deuteronomy 8:2–3).

If God has me in the wilderness, it's because He is preparing, strengthening, and refining me for something greater. This isn't punishment—it's spiritual training.

Sometimes we think God is delaying, when in reality He's developing us. The silence, the waiting, the unanswered prayers—they're not signs of His absence but the soil where endurance, humility, and faith take root.

The wilderness becomes the laboratory of the Spirit— where emotional storms meet divine order. It's where the Mind of the Spirit begins to form within us, creating a gap between reaction and response,[28] teaching us to breathe with

---

[28] DBT teaches individuals to slow down automatic reactions through

God instead of breaking beneath the waiting. As Scripture says, "Be still, and know that I am God" (Psalm 46:10).

When everything in our adoption case was spinning again—emails from social workers, new court dates—I felt my chest tighten before I even knew what was wrong. Sometimes, early in the morning before anyone was up, I would just sit in silence before God in tears, whispering, "Okay, God, I'm here." It wasn't peaceful; it was raw. But sitting there without fixing anything felt like the tiniest act of worship, proof that I could stay present in the ache instead of running from it.

Radical Acceptance: The Doorway to Divine Strength

In DBT, the foundation of Distress Tolerance is Radical Acceptance[29]—fully acknowledging what is, without resistance or denial. It doesn't mean approval; it means surrendering to God my reality[30] so His peace can begin

---

mindfulness, widening the space between trigger and action to allow wise, value-aligned choices (Linehan 2015).

[29] Radical Acceptance is the DBT practice of fully acknowledging reality without judgment or resistance, which reduces suffering caused by fighting unchangeable circumstances (Linehan 2015).

[30] DBT distinguishes acceptance from agreement—acceptance means acknowledging what is true, not condoning it (Hayes et al. 1999; Linehan 2015).

to enter. Acceptance names reality truthfully; it does not excuse injustice, silence grief, or require us to stop longing for change.

Radical Acceptance for me usually happens with a tooth-brush in one hand and tears in my eyes. I'll catch myself trying to control the narrative again—rehearsing what to say to the attorney, the social worker, my friends, and even myself. Then I stop and remind myself to stay curious: *This is my wilderness today. How might God be preparing me?* I turn my attention from control to awe and curiosity about what God might be doing.

It doesn't change the facts, but it changes the fight inside me.

Spiritually, Radical Acceptance sounds like saying, "This is hard. This hurts. I wish it were different—but God, You are still good."

Before God can prepare us for something greater, He often strips away the illusion of control. The Israelites had to learn dependence on manna before they could inherit the Promised Land. Jesus had to endure hunger before feeding others with eternal bread. Paul had to lose his status before he could gain true authority.

When I stopped fighting the reality that I was in the wilderness, and stopped asking *"How do I get out?"*, I began asking a new question, *"What are You forming in me here?"* That question became the beginning of peace.

Abraham: Radical Acceptance Empowered by Promise

Abraham's story in Romans 4 shows what Radical Acceptance looks like when it's infused with supernatural faith. He lived in the wilderness between *promise* and *fulfillment*, facing the painful reality that his body was "as good as dead," yet choosing to believe that God could still bring life from what seemed impossible.

> Against all hope, Abraham in hope believed . . . Without weakening in his faith, he faced the fact that his body was as good as dead . . . Yet he did not waver through unbelief regarding the promise of God, but was strengthened in his faith and gave glory to God, being fully persuaded that God had power to do what He had promised. (v. 18-21)

Abraham's acceptance wasn't passive resignation—it was active faith. He faced the facts but kept believing that God could "call into being things that were not."

That's the essence of spiritual Radical Acceptance:

- Facing reality without denying the pain.
- Holding faith without demanding control.
- Trusting that what feels dead is often the soil of resurrection.

When we accept what is with eyes of faith, we become strengthened like Abraham, fully persuaded that God still has power to do what He has promised. This kind of acceptance doesn't weaken faith; it anchors it. It gives suffering context and keeps us from being consumed by despair, because even when nothing changes today, God is still working beneath the surface for tomorrow.

I relate to Abraham's waiting more than I ever wanted to. I've looked at situations that felt dead—relationships, court decisions, even my own hope of having a family—and heard God whisper, *"Stay."* Some nights, I caught myself preoccupied, worrying about what could happen, and I had to stop and remind myself to be present in the moment. I didn't know how much longer I would have with our boys, but I knew God was still sovereign—even when I had no control, and even when the outcome remained uncertain.

Realizing this allowed me to slow down and truly enjoy them—to watch their favorite cartoons, prepare chocolate milk, sing songs, teach them to ride bikes, and hold them close at bedtime. Hope, for me, isn't optimism; it's showing up with open hands even when my heart feels afraid.

Self-Soothing and Whole Integration: Living Through the Spirit

The wilderness strips away external comforts, but it also teaches us the holy art of living through the Spirit in the middle of suffering.

DBT calls this *self-soothing*—engaging the senses to calm the body[31] when the mind feels unsafe. Spiritually, it's deeper than coping; it's communion. It's learning to let God meet us in the ordinary rhythms of being human.

When we practice Radical Acceptance, we begin to reclaim our ability to function. Instead of collapsing into despair, we start participating in life again. We do the small, steady things—eating, resting, showering, showing up—because we still hope even while we radically accept what is. These Activities of Daily Living[32] become acts of faith, small "yeses" to life when everything in us wants to give up and surrender to the Mind of the Flesh rather than to the Mind of the Spirit.

Some evenings, when my thoughts won't stop spiraling, I put on my AirPods, turn on Christian salsa music, and start washing the dishes. The warm water, the scent of soap, the rhythm in my ears—it calms my nervous system in a way prayer alone sometimes can't. I let the lyrics preach to me while my hands move. Sometimes I shed a quiet tear; other times, I smile at a memory that surfaces.

---

[31] Self-soothing is a Distress Tolerance skill that uses sensory experiences (touch, sound, taste, smell, sight) to calm physiological arousal and promote emotional grounding (Linehan 2015).

[32] DBT encourages engaging in simple behavioral actions (e.g., eating, bathing, completing routine tasks) to stabilize functioning during distress, known as "improving the moment" and crisis survival (Linehan 2015).

That small act of engagement—moving my body, listening, remembering, worshiping—grounds me again. In those moments of music, motion, and soap bubbles, the noise in my mind softens enough for me to sense God near.

That's what integration looks like in my kitchen: DBT and theology meeting dishwater.

This is where integration happens—where the spiritual meets the physical, and we become whole. God designed us as both spirit and body, each needing care. Our surrender and self-care become acts of obedience. When we make the bed, breathe deeply, go for a walk, or eat a meal with gratitude, we aren't abandoning our spiritual life—we're embodying it.

Every small act of care becomes communion with God:

- Eating when grief dulls your appetite becomes trust: *God will sustain me.*

- Getting out of bed becomes a declaration: *Life is still worth living.*

- Brushing your teeth, folding laundry, lighting a candle—all become embodied prayers that whisper, *I am still here. God is still with me.*

In these moments, the Spirit inhabits our breath, our senses, our ordinary rhythms, until peace moves from concept to incarnation—Christ alive in us.

Choosing to self-soothe and engage in acts of daily living has become my way of overcoming. Where the Mind of the Flesh or Emotion Mind urges me to give up, the Mind of the

Spirit—focused on God's promises—enables me to move forward and participate in life. It does this despite the pain and urges of emotional distress. This is where breakthroughs are born. This is where God grows me beyond comfort and teaches me to live skillfully, even when I fail trying.

These small acts became lifelines. Over time, they shifted from coping to communion with God. They weren't just ways to get through the day—they became ways to experience God *in* the day, as a whole integrated being: body, mind, and spirit held together by grace. The wilderness doesn't tell us why God allows suffering—but it teaches us how God remains present within it.

From Distress to Destiny

I used to think practicing these skills would make me calm—or maybe appear "normal." Now I know they help me stay connected when I'm not calm, and that this messy, human experience *is* normal.

Distress Tolerance for me means choosing not to shut down in the waiting, not to scroll endlessly on my phone, not to chase control. It's breathing, naming what's real, and trusting that God hasn't left me alone in the wilderness.

Eventually, I began to see that every moment of distress tolerance was really a moment of spiritual formation.[33] The

---

[33] Distress Tolerance practices strengthen long-term resilience by training

wilderness wasn't meant to destroy me—it was meant to develop me.

Each breath, each act of acceptance, each ordinary moment of perseverance was quietly preparing me for the life God was calling me to carry.

Just as Jesus left the wilderness "in the power of the Spirit" (Luke 4:14), we too emerge stronger, more centered, and more aware of the God who sustains us.

The wilderness is not wasted. It is worship. It's where distress becomes dialogue with God, and waiting becomes witness to His refining love.

I'm still learning this. Some days I light my own fires again;[34] some days I actually rest. But even in my relapses back into these unhealthy ways of coping, I can feel the Spirit inviting me back—not to performance, but to Presence.

Pause and Practice

Scripture Meditation

"Wait for the Lord; be strong and take heart and wait for the Lord" (Psalm 27:14).

---

both emotional and cognitive systems to remain regulated despite intense discomfort (Linehan 2015; Lynch 2018).

[34] DBT conceptualizes relapse into old coping patterns as a normal part of skill acquisition, emphasizing returning to mindfulness rather than self-criticism (Linehan 2015).

Surrender Prayer

"Lord, I accept what is before me, trusting that Your love is still working beneath what I cannot see. Teach me to wait without panic, to suffer without despair, and to find You in the space between my pain and Your promise."

Gentle Practice

When distress rises, pause.

Breathe deeply.

Do one small thing that honors your body and spirit—eat, walk, pray, or rest.

Let that act become your declaration:*I am still here, and so is God.*

Closing Thought

The wilderness will always feel uncomfortable—but it no longer has to feel empty. Every time we choose to wait with God rather than run from Him, something spiritual takes root in us.

The same Spirit who led Jesus into the desert leads us also—not to destroy us, but to prepare us. Distress Tolerance isn't just a therapy skill; it's a spiritual posture. And when we learn to sit in the wilderness with God, we discover that endurance itself becomes encounter.

CHAPTER 5

Emotion Regulation: Letting the Spirit Rule the Heart

If Chapter 4 asks how we stay with God when we cannot change our circumstances, this chapter asks how we steward what is happening *inside* us while we wait. When circumstances remain unresolved, what often becomes most urgent is what is happening inside us. Chapter 5 turns toward the inner life—exploring how emotions can either pull us out of God's presence or become places of return, repentance, and renewed alignment with the Spirit.

What Is Emotion Regulation?In DBT, *Emotion Regulation*[35] is the foundational skill set that helps us understand, organize, and influence our emotional experience so we are

---

[35] Emotion Regulation in DBT refers to skills that help individuals identify, understand, and modify emotional responses in ways that reduce vulnerability and increase long-term well-being (Linehan 2015).

no longer ruled by overpowering feelings. It teaches us how to identify what we feel, reduce emotional vulnerability, shift emotional intensity, and make wise, grounded choices even when our inner world feels chaotic. Emotion Regulation isn't about "controlling" emotions; it's about restoring balance so emotions can guide us rather than overwhelm us.

Spiritually, Emotion Regulation is the practice of aligning our inner life with the presence of God. It is the journey of learning to recognize what is happening inside us—fear, anger, hope, grief—and inviting the Holy Spirit into that space. It's choosing to respond from the Mind of the Spirit rather than the Mind of the Flesh, allowing the fruit of the Spirit to shape our emotional lives instead of letting unprocessed feelings dictate our reactions.

Emotion Regulation is not the absence of emotion; it is the integration of emotion with wisdom, compassion, and divine presence. It is the slow, holy work of becoming people whose hearts are steady even in storms—not because we feel less, but because we walk with God through what we feel. A steady heart does not prevent storms from forming—it keeps us from becoming the storm that harms ourselves or others.

The Heart as the Battleground

When I was twenty-three, I learned how fierce the battle inside the heart can be. That year, I had been diagnosed with complex PTSD and was beginning to face the trauma I'd carried since childhood. I thought the worst was behind me—until a doctor found a strange bulge in the back of my throat. He asked quietly, "Is there a history of young people with cancer in your family?"

A CT scan and MRI confirmed a large tumor—roughly the size of a lemon—pressing into my brainstem. It had already cut off circulation to my left jugular vein, wrapped around my carotid artery, and paralyzed my left vocal cord. We were seeking medical opinions, and a surgeon at University of California, San Francisco Medical Center told me, "It isn't a question of whether you survive the surgery; it's about what quality of life you'll have afterward." He warned I might lose the ability to eat or breathe on my own, that I could need a permanent tracheotomy and feeding tube, or even lose part of my skull. And before they operated, they wouldn't know if the tumor was cancerous.

While processing all this, I was working full-time as a credit counselor in San Francisco—helping families avoid bankruptcy. Nine out of ten of my clients were drowning because of medical debt. One woman had gone blind and depended on her seven-year-old daughter to read her statements aloud. Another had cancer and could no longer work. As I counseled them through their crises, I was quietly living one of my own. Between phone sessions, I'd cry in the break room or slip outside, put on my headphones, and blast Matisyahu's Album *One Day*—songs of hope, faith, and defiant praise.

Sometimes those walks down Market Street became my sanctuary. Other times, I drove to Rockaway Beach in

Pacifica, climbed the cliffs, and screamed prayers into the wind. It wasn't pretty prayer. It was *ugly*, guttural, and soaked in tears. I would ask, "Is this it, God? Twenty-three years—is that all I get? Will I never get married? Will I never have a family?"

My emotions were a storm—fear, rage, bargaining, despair. I wanted to numb out so badly. I'd never been into alcohol, but suddenly I wanted to get drunk, to feel nothing. Part of me even considered reckless hookups just to forget the terror for a night. Deep down, I knew those temptations were false comforts. These impulses weren't explicit efforts to rebel against God; they were distress signals in a nervous system searching for relief, when I doubted God's desire and ability to comfort me in the way I needed most. I needed to take my doubts to God. I stayed sober, stayed guarded, and chose instead to face the pain head-on with God.

That decision—to *feel* instead of flee[36]—was my first step into what DBT calls emotion-regulation and what Scripture describes as surrender.

I began naming[37] every emotion before God instead of hiding it: anger, fear, grief, loneliness, envy of the healthy

---

[36] DBT emphasizes allowing emotional experience rather than suppressing or avoiding it, as avoidance amplifies distress and prevents emotional processing (Hayes et al. 1999; Linehan 2015).

[37] Identifying and labeling emotions ("Name it to tame it") is a DBT strategy shown to reduce emotional intensity and increase prefrontal cortex regulation (Linehan 2015; Siegel 2012).

people walking past me. I learned that emotions, like waves, lose power when they are brought into the light.

There on the cliffs at Rockaway Beach, I gave God every feeling I had, and something miraculous happened. Once I stopped pretending, the Spirit met me in the mess. The anger that once roared became a whisper of peace. In that surrender, I heard a deeper truth: "Even if life ends at twenty-three, I am still enough."

Romans 12:1–2 became real to me, ". . . offer your bodies as a living sacrifice . . . Then you will be able to test and approve what God's will is—His good, pleasing and perfect will."

That day, I offered God not just my body but my emotions—the rawest parts of me. I accepted that whatever His will was, it would be good, pleasing, and perfect, even if it cost me everything. That surrender did not mean approving of suffering; it meant trusting God's presence even when the outcome remained uncertain.

When I finally climbed down from the cliffs, my circumstances hadn't changed. The tumor was still there. The surgery still loomed. But the *battle inside my heart* had shifted. I came down ready for whatever came next. I wasn't fearless—but I was no longer ruled by fear.

That's when I first understood what it means to let the Spirit rule the heart.

Emotion didn't disappear—it found its rightful place under divine authority. Peace didn't erase pain—it transformed it.

These days, emotion regulation looks less like cliff-side surrender and more like micro-surrenders. When I feel overwhelmed—by work, marriage, foster parenting, or uncertainty with my health—I pause and name what's true: *I'm afraid.* Then I breathe, recall a verse, and invite the Spirit to sit with me. The goal isn't to make the fear disappear; it's to stay connected to God inside it. Sometimes peace feels like stillness, and other times it just feels like not running away.

The Fruit of the Spirit—Embracing Emotional Surrender

When I look back on that season, I can see that the Spirit wasn't only healing my body—He was renewing my mind. Before surgery, my prayers were desperate and raw, but afterward they became quieter, more reflective. Something had shifted.

The Holy Spirit began teaching me what both Scripture and psychology affirm: emotional maturity is born through surrender, not control.

In DBT, this process is called *Radical Acceptance*[38]—acknowledging reality without judgment or resistance while still holding space for hope and change. Scripture calls it

[38] Radical Acceptance is used both in Distress Tolerance and Emotion Regulation to help individuals accept internal experience without judgment while committing to value-aligned action (Linehan 2015).

faith—trusting that even when we can't see or fix the outcome, God is working all things together for good (Romans 8:28).

I had spent years trying to perfect myself, to be strong, to manage my emotions through effort and discipline. But in the face of my brain tumor, all that self-sufficiency shattered. I couldn't control anything—not my body, not the future, not even the shape of my own prayers. Yet it was there I learned the paradox Paul spoke of: "My grace is sufficient for you, for My power is made perfect in weakness" (2 Corinthians 12:9).

Weakness became liberation. The more I admitted my need, the freer I became. In DBT terms, I was moving from Emotion Mind—where fear ruled—to Wise Mind—where truth and emotion found balance under the Spirit's rule.

As I practiced Radical Acceptance in prayer—naming my emotions honestly before God—I found that peace was not the absence of pain but the presence of divine alignment. Just as the prophet Isaiah says, "You will keep in perfect peace those whose minds are steadfast, because they trust in You" (Isaiah 26:3).

Peace came when I stopped fighting my humanity. It came when I could say, "God, I am helpless—and that's okay," because helplessness was no longer a threat to my identity. It was an invitation for God's power to rest on me.

Slowly, I began to see that emotions were not obstacles to faith—they were invitations to transformation. Now, whenever I feel defensive or hurt in conversation[39] I try to pause and listen before reacting. Instead of shutting down, I ask myself, *What is this emotion trying to tell me?* Sometimes it reveals pride, insecurity, bitterness; other times, exhaustion or fear—or all of it tangled together.

When I bring that awareness into prayer, the Spirit begins to soften what was hard and steady what was scattered. That's when emotion becomes a bridge instead of a barrier—when pain becomes a teacher, sadness becomes holy ground for comfort, and weakness becomes the doorway to humility and deeper intimacy with God.

DBT teaches that emotions have purpose[40]—they signal our needs, our values, and our limits. Scripture agrees. The psalmists didn't hide their emotions; they sanctified them through expression. For example, Psalm 56:3 says, "When I am afraid, I put my trust in You."

David's honesty wasn't unspiritual—it was holy. That's what the Spirit was doing in me: turning raw emotion into revelation, chaos into communion.

I began to understand Jesus's invitation: "Blessed are those who mourn, for they will be comforted" (Matthew 5:4).

---

[39] Opposite Action is a DBT Emotion Regulation strategy in which individuals act opposite to emotional urges when those emotions do not fit the facts or are unhelpful (Linehan 2015).

[40] According to DBT, emotions function to motivate action, communicate with others, and communicate to oneself important information about needs and values (Linehan 2015).

That comfort isn't passive; it's the fruit of emotional surrender—of letting God comfort us instead of numbing ourselves.

I started to see that my worth wasn't in my performance or stability. Confidence in those things counted for nothing; confidence in God's presence counted for everything.

In DBT, this is called *Building Mastery*[41]—learning to act from effectiveness, not emotion. Spiritually, it means living from our identity in Christ, not insecurity.

As I practiced this, the fruits of the Spirit from Galatians 5 began to grow in places where anxiety once lived: love instead of self-protection, peace instead of panic, patience instead of perfectionism, self-control instead of shame.

Healing was painful—but it was holy pain, the kind that transforms. Weakness wasn't failure—it was freedom. Pain didn't define me—it refined me. Peace didn't come by control—it came by surrender.

The Spirit was teaching me, in language both psychological and holy, that true emotional regulation is not suppression—it's Spirit-led integration. As Romans 8:6 says, ". . . the mind governed by the Spirit is life and peace."

---

[41] Building Mastery is an Emotion Regulation skill involving daily actions that increase competence and reduce helplessness by engaging in activities aligned with one's values (Linehan 2015).

When Disconnection Becomes the Real Distress: Understanding Sin Through Emotional Regulation

The more I studied both Scripture and psychology, the clearer it became that emotional regulation isn't only about calming down—it's about staying connected and integrated into God's will and His Kingdom.

When emotions spin out of control, our instinct is to reach for relief. The Mind of the Flesh (Emotion Mind) craves comfort; the Mind of the World (Reason Mind) craves control. Both are desperate to fill the inner void that forms when we drift out of alignment with the Spirit and outside of God's will for His Kingdom.

When I get flooded—especially during stressful updates about our case, tight deadlines at work, conflict in marriage, or my ongoing battles with mental and physical health—I can feel my brain start scrambling for control. I want to email or text someone, fix something, prove I'm doing enough. But lately, I've started pausing instead of performing.[42] I take a walk, talk to God out loud, or sit on the couch with my coffee until the urgency settles. Those small pauses keep me tethered to peace instead of panic.

In moments like these, I realize that emotional reactivity isn't just stress—it's a form of spiritual disconnection.

---

[42] Emotion Regulation includes reducing vulnerability to emotional intensity by addressing factors such as sleep, nutrition, illness, stress, and substance use—known as the ABC PLEASE skills (Linehan 2015).

When I reach for control instead of communion, I'm stepping out of alignment with the Spirit, His good, pleasing, and perfect will for how I am meant to live within His Kingdom. Naming this misalignment is not self-accusation; it is the beginning of agreement with God, repentance, and repair.

That disconnection—between our heart and God's presence—is what Scripture calls sin.

Not merely moral failure, but misalignment between ourselves and God's Spirit. Not just doing wrong, but acting—or failing to act—outside of love, truth, the example of Jesus and God's will for His Kingdom.

When we sin, we step away from God's Spirit of peace, from the living water meant to fill us. That void aches to be filled. The Mind of the Flesh tries to fill it with false comforts—impulse, empty pleasure, distraction, addiction, comparison. The Mind of the World tries to fill it with reasoning and control—"If I can just understand this, I'll feel safe again."

But neither Flesh nor World can satisfy the thirst for the Spirit.

On the last and greatest day of the festival, Jesus stood and said in a loud voice, 'Let anyone who is thirsty come to me and drink. Whoever believes in me, as Scripture has said, rivers of living water will flow from within them.' By this he meant the Spirit . . . (John 7:37-39)

Emotional dysregulation often signals this thirst. When I become reactive, numb, or spiritually dry, it's rarely just about my circumstances—it's about my disconnection. I've stepped outside of alignment with my biblical values, even if it was unintentional.

In DBT, this is the moment for non-judgmental awareness—to observe the behavior, name it, and gently return to center. Spiritually, this is called repentance—not condemnation, but conviction; it is my *realignment* with my biblical values.

Repentance is the art of coming back to the presence of God. It's when we stop running, stop reasoning, and begin seeking God's will, Kingdom, and agree to let the Spirit fill the empty spaces again.

In DBT, emotion regulation is maintained through *mindfulness*—staying aware of our internal states without judging them. In Scripture, it's the call to *"Be still and know that I am God"* (Psalm 46:10). When we notice our impulses, our emotional reactions, and the ways we're trying to self-soothe apart from God, we can confess, "Lord, I've stepped outside of trusting your good, pleasing and perfect will. I am sorry, help me come back again," and return to His presence.

That's how we course-correct spiritually. We don't fix ourselves—we confess, we recognize God's goodness, and we *return* to Him. As we return, the living water flows again. Peace replaces panic. Presence replaces striving.

This is where emotional regulation becomes spiritual formation:

- DBT teaches us to observe without judgment.[43] Scripture teaches us to *repent without shame.*[44]

- DBT helps us build skillful responses. Scripture convicts us and helps us *walk in the Spirit* (Galatians 5:16).

- DBT grounds us in the present moment. Scripture grounds us in God's will and presence—the living water that restores the soul.

When we notice our sin—our misalignment—with compassion and conviction, rather than condemnation, we can re-enter God's presence sooner. And the more we return to God's presence, the less we will act from the Emotion Mind or Reason Mind. As Galatians says, "If we live by the Spirit, let us also keep in step with the Spirit" (5:25).

---

[43] Mindfulness practices help individuals regulate emotions by increasing awareness of internal states and decreasing reactivity (Bishop et al. 2004; Linehan 2015).

[44] DBT emphasizes non-judgmental awareness and skillful return to center when dysregulated—a parallel to spiritual practices of confession and re-alignment (Linehan 2015; Hayes et al. 2011).

Summary Reflection:
Sin and the Mind of the Spirit[45]

Concept	Mind of the Flesh / Emotion Mind	Mind of the World / Reason Mind	Mind of the Spirit / Wise Mind
Core Desire	Comfort	Control	Connection
Coping Pattern	Impulsivity, numbing, indulgence	Overthinking, striving, detachment	Conviction, surrender, prayer, repentance
Result	Shame & exhaustion	Pride & anxiety	Peace & alignment
Spiritual Parallel	"Drinking from broken cisterns" *(Jer 2:13)*	"Leaning on your own understanding" *(Prov 3:5)*	"Streams of living water" *(John 7:38)*

The goal isn't perfection—it's presence.

---

[45] DBT describes three core mind states—Emotion Mind, Reason Mind, and Wise Mind—representing emotional reactivity, cognitive analysis, and integrated awareness, respectively (Linehan 2015).

To keep walking, repenting, and realigning with the Spirit who fills every void that other comforts leave empty.

When the Spirit Rules the Heart

The more I practiced returning to God's presence, the more I discovered that the Spirit doesn't erase emotion; He *restores* it. Restoring emotions means the Spirit conforms our hearts to God's values and will.

When the Spirit rules the heart:

- Anger becomes mercy.
- Sadness becomes hope.
- Fear becomes trust.
- Guilt becomes gratitude.

Letting the Spirit rule the heart[46] doesn't make us less human—it makes us fully able to experience the peace God offers in John 14:27, "Peace I leave with you; my peace I give you. I do not give to you as the world gives. Do not let your hearts be troubled and do not be afraid."

That peace isn't passive; it's active, like a guard standing watch over our inner world. It doesn't silence emotion; it purifies it.

---

[46] Wise Mind is the DBT state of emotional balance, clarity, and value-aligned action—integrating both emotional truth and grounded thinking (Linehan 2015).

The same Spirit who calmed me on those cliffs in Pacifica still whispers through every emotional storm: *"You don't have to be unfeeling to be faithful. You just have to let Me lead."*

Reflection and Practice

Scripture Meditation

> "Let the peace of Christ rule in your hearts, since as members of one body you were called to peace. And be thankful" (Colossians 3:15).

Peace isn't something we achieve; it's given to us by God when we allow the Spirit to rule.

When we have conflict in our hearts—fear versus faith, anger versus compassion, despair versus hope—the Spirit becomes the umpire who calls what's true and what's out of bounds.

Ask yourself:

- Which emotion has been trying to rule my heart lately?
- What truth might the Spirit be inviting me to see?
- What would it look like to let the Spirit call the play?

Prayer of Return – When Emotions Are Loud

God,
I feel overwhelmed, reactive, or disconnected right now.
I don't want to run, numb, control, or fix myself apart from You.

I acknowledge where my emotions are leading me away from
Your love, Your will, and Your Kingdom,
I am tempted and/or acting out away from truth and away
from Your presence.

I am convicted, but not condemned.
I'm here to come back to obedience—obedience that flows
from Your will, Your love, and Your Kingdom.

I return to You—
to Your Spirit,
to Your presence,
to Your good and gentle Kingdom rule in my heart.

Fill the empty places again.
Quiet what is frantic.
Soften what is hard.
Strengthen what is weary.

Let Your Spirit rule my heart
so my pain does not become harmful to myself or others,
and my emotions serve you in love instead of fear.

I choose communion with You over control.
Your presence over performance.
Return over retreat.
In Jesus Name, Amen.

Journal Prompt

- When you feel emotionally overwhelmed, where are you most tempted to disconnect—from God, from others, or from yourself?

- What behaviors or patterns tend to emerge in those moments? (Avoid judgment here; simply name what happens.)

- How might returning to God's presence in that moment interrupt the passing of pain forward—to yourself or to others?

- What would obedience to love look like right there, even if the emotion doesn't immediately change?

Closing Thought

Emotion regulation in the Mind of the Spirit is not emotional control—it's emotional communion. It's learning to bring our humanity to God's holiness.

When the Spirit rules the heart, emotions are no longer enemies of faith—they become instruments of worship. We feel deeply, love bravely, and live peacefully—not because the storm stops, but because the Spirit sits in the driver's seat.

CHAPTER 6

Speaking the Truth in Love: Interpersonal Effectiveness Under the Rule of the Kingdom

If Chapters 4 and 5 shape how we endure and regulate under God's rule, this chapter asks how that inner alignment is lived out in community—through truth, boundaries, and love. When we have learned to endure with God and tend to our inner world under His rule, the question inevitably turns outward: how do we live this faith with other people? This chapter explores what it means to speak the truth in love—through boundaries, responsibility, and reconciliation shaped by the order of God's Kingdom.

What Is Interpersonal Effectiveness?In DBT, *Interpersonal Effectiveness* is the ability to navigate relationships[47]

---

[47] Interpersonal Effectiveness in DBT consists of skills that help individuals advocate for their needs, maintain healthy relationships, and act

with clarity, honesty, and integrity. It teaches us how to ask for what we need, set boundaries without shame, maintain connection without losing ourselves, and communicate truth without sacrificing compassion. At its core, it is relational wisdom—the skill of balancing three essential goals: getting our needs met,[48] preserving the relationship, and protecting our self-respect.

Interpersonal Effectiveness isn't about winning arguments or avoiding conflict. It's about communicating in a way that reflects our values, honors our identity, and builds genuine connection. It helps us move out of fear, silence, people-pleasing, or defensiveness and into grounded, confident, Spirit-aligned presence.

Spiritually, Interpersonal Effectiveness is the practice of loving others the way Jesus loved—with grace that never abandons truth and truth that never abandons love. It's the courage to speak honestly, to listen humbly, and to stay connected even in discomfort. It is the sacred work of letting the Spirit guide our voice, soften our tone, and anchor our identity so fear no longer governs our relationships.

Interpersonal Effectiveness teaches us to communicate not from the Mind of the Flesh—reactive, fearful,

---

in alignment with their values during interpersonal exchanges (Linehan 2015).

[48] DBT organizes interpersonal skills around three core aims: Objective Effectiveness, Relationship Effectiveness, and Self-Respect Effectiveness (Linehan 2015).

self-protective—but from the Mind of the Spirit, where truth and love walk hand in hand. It is the relational expression of spiritual maturity: learning to show up honestly, humbly, and courageously in the presence of others, even when our voice trembles.

Jesus did not pray for our comfort.

On the night before His crucifixion, He prayed for our unity.

> "I pray that they will all be one, just as You and I are one . . . so that the world may believe that You sent Me" (John 17:21).

This prayer is not sentimental. Jesus ties the credibility of the gospel to the *visible life of His people*. Unity, in Scripture, is not sameness, emotional harmony, or avoidance of conflict. It is a *shared submission to God's will*, lived out through truth, love, responsibility, and ordered relationships.

For much of my life, I misunderstood this. I believed unity meant staying agreeable, staying available, and staying quiet when truth felt risky. I wanted peace so badly that I confused silence with love and emotional restraint with faithfulness. Over time, I learned that this kind of peace does not build the Kingdom—it erodes it quietly.

Unity in the Kingdom is not accidental.

It is cultivated.

And it has order.

The Command That Governs the Kingdom

On the same night He prayed for unity, Jesus gave His disciples a command:

> "So I give you now a new commandment: Love each other just as much as I have loved you. For when you demonstrate the same love I have for you by loving one another, everyone will know that you're my true followers" (John 13:34–35, TPT).

Jesus does not define love by emotional comfort, mutual understanding, or relational success. He defines it by His own way of loving—truthful, sacrificial, having boundaries, and being obedient to the Father.

This reframes everything.

Love in the Kingdom is not measured by how little conflict we create, but by how faithfully we reflect God's truth and character *within* relationship. Speaking the truth in love is not optional maturity—it is obedience.

Jesus, Solitude, and Alignment Before Engagement

Jesus desired unity deeply, but He never pursued it through over-functioning or boundarylessness.

Again and again, Scripture shows Him withdrawing to solitary places to pray (Mark 1:35; Luke 5:16)—often when people were actively demanding His presence. Before engaging others, Jesus aligned with the Father.

This pattern reshaped my understanding of boundaries.

In moments of relational tension, my instinct has often been urgency—to explain, to fix, to clarify, to restore connection immediately. But when I speak from urgency, my words carry anxiety rather than love. I have learned, often through regret, that alignment must come before engagement.

Withdrawal to pray is not avoidance.

It is obedience.

Boundaries are not withdrawal from love; they are alignment with God, so love can be rightly ordered.

Interpersonal Effectiveness Under a Kingdom Arch

DBT's Interpersonal Effectiveness module identifies three core objectives:

1. Objective Effectiveness – getting legitimate needs met

2. Relationship Effectiveness – preserving the relationship

3. Self-Respect Effectiveness – maintaining integrity and values

These objectives are biblically consistent—but they are not ultimate.

In the Kingdom of God, interpersonal effectiveness serves a higher aim: that God's will would be done, His character reflected, and His people formed into maturity.

Kingdom-Level Objective (Overarching All Others)

To speak and act in ways that reflect God's truth, love, and order so that His Kingdom is made visible on earth as it is in heaven.

DBT skills are not the goal. They are servants of formation.

Interpersonal Effectiveness Reframed Under the Kingdom

Kingdom Aim	DBT Expression
Faithfulness to truth	Objective Effectiveness
Preservation of the Body	Relationship Effectiveness
Integrity before God	Self-Respect Effectiveness

This matters because speaking the truth in love is not about emotional discharge, persuasion, or control. It is about faithfulness—naming reality without judgment and releasing outcomes to God.

Truth, Love, and Responsibility in the Body of Christ

Scripture describes the Church as a living body, "closely joined together and constantly connected as one" (Ephesians 4:16). Each member has a responsibility. No one carries everything. But everyone carries something.

Galatians 6 makes this distinction explicit:

- "Carry each other's burdens . . ." (verse 2)
- "Each one should carry their own load." (verse 5)

Burdens are crushing weights—grief, suffering, injustice.

Loads are personal responsibilities—our words, choices, repentance, and obedience.

Confusing these leads either to abandonment or enmeshment—neither of which reflects the Kingdom.

Where I Have Failed to Live This Faithfully

I need to name this honestly—not as self-condemnation, but as clarity.

There have been times I crossed others' boundaries by seeking from them what I was meant to carry to God. I over-texted. I vented repeatedly. I processed my pain externally before submitting it internally to the Spirit. At times, I used vulnerability to discharge emotion rather than to seek wisdom or repair.

When others could not meet those needs—or offered boundaries instead of reassurance—I felt hurt or bitter. I analyzed my trauma. I named my triggers. I explained my pain. All of that mattered. But I did not always take responsibility for how I coped with that pain.

There were also times I resisted influence. Pride disguised itself as clarity. I wanted understanding without repentance, validation without surrender, comfort without change.

This is where sin becomes uncomfortable to name—not because trauma isn't real, but because there are ways of coping with pain that move me outside God's will and the culture of His Kingdom.

Owning this does not mean I carry full responsibility for relational breakdown. In the Kingdom, responsibility is shared. I cannot control others, and I cannot use emotion—whether silence or intensity—to manipulate them into responsibility.

Speaking the truth in love means stating the facts without judgment, naming my responsibility clearly, and entrusting the outcome to God.

A Personal Reckoning: When Presence Is Not Yet Obedience

Most mornings, my body wakes up before my mind is ready.

Between three and four a.m., I often jolt awake from nightmares—my nervous system already flooded with fear before I've had a chance to orient myself to the present. The house is quiet. The world is still asleep. But inside me, everything is loud.

I do what I know to do. I regulate my breathing. I ground myself in the present moment. I open my Bible. I journal. Some mornings I sit with Scripture for nearly two hours, from four until six, praying, reading, writing, listening. I am not avoiding God. I am not ignoring Him.

And still, there are mornings when I remain deeply unsettled.

Sometimes the quiet brings conviction—clarity about sin, character, or misalignment. Other times it turns inward, becoming anxiety, fear, or self-accusation. I know the truth. I can quote Scripture. And yet my body is still activated, my thoughts still racing, my distress still high.

This is where I've had to face a harder truth: being with God is not the same as doing the good I know to do.

James writes, "If anyone knows the good they ought to do and doesn't do it, it is sin" (James 4:17). I used to think of sin primarily as doing what I shouldn't. I am learning that it also includes not doing what love, wisdom, and obedience require.

There are mornings when what is missing is not more prayer, but participation.

I have DBT tools I know how to use—distress tolerance skills, radical acceptance, grounding through movement, engaging my senses, and allowing emotion to rise and fall without acting on it. I know the importance of daily acts of living: eating, moving my body, taking my medication consistently, and caring for my physical health. These are not secondary to faith. They are part of the load God has entrusted to me.

And yet, in my desperation, I sometimes skip these steps.

Instead of tolerating distress, I flee from it.

Instead of accepting what I cannot change in that moment, I fight it.

Instead of caring for my body, I dissociate from it.

I know the good I ought to do—and I don't always do it. That is often the moment when I reach for my phone.

Between five and six a.m., I begin typing long, emotionally intense messages to friends who are just waking up or preparing for their own time with God. Paragraphs spill out—fear, insight, despair, urgency. I call it honesty. I call it asking for help. But often, it is bypassing the slow, embodied obedience God is inviting me into.

I am not wrong to need help. The Body of Christ is real, and Scripture calls us to bear one another's burdens. But what I am learning is that help must be sought within order.

Friends are not meant to replace distress tolerance.

They are not meant to absorb unprocessed urgency.

They are not meant to be awakened into crises that God is inviting me to endure faithfully.

When I reach for others before I have fully carried my own load—before eating, before moving, before taking medication, before practicing the skills I know—I unintentionally ask them to carry what God has already equipped me to steward.

This is not a failure of desire. It is a failure of integration.

God's Kingdom is not only entered through prayer; it is lived through obedience in small, embodied ways. Sometimes faithfulness looks like sitting with distress a little longer. Sometimes it looks like waiting until daylight to ask for support. Sometimes it looks like sending a short, respectful message instead of an emotional flood: *I'm having a hard morning. Can we talk later today?*

That is still asking for help.

But it is asking within order.

I am learning that God often wants to carry my load through daily faithfulness, not instead of it. And when I do that—when I tolerate distress, accept reality, care for my body, and honor boundaries—my need for others becomes clearer, calmer, and more mutual.

Friends are then able to support me as members of the Body, not as emergency responders to pain I have not yet stewarded.

Paul names this conflict with brutal honesty in Romans 7. He describes knowing the good he ought to do and still finding himself doing the opposite—not because he lacks desire or knowledge, but because something within him resists alignment. Romans 7 does not deny responsibility; it explains the depth of our need. It names the tension between intention and action, conviction and follow-through. And it refuses the fantasy that insight alone is enough. Paul's answer is not despair or resignation, but deliverance: "Thanks be to God, who delivers me through Jesus Christ our Lord" (Romans 7:25).

Integrating DBT Skills When Distress Persists

When God has been sought and distress remains, faithfulness often requires participation, not more insight.

Distress Tolerance

Staying present without acting impulsively (TIPP, grounding, radical acceptance) is obedience when emotions demand urgency.

Emotion Regulation

PLEASE skills—sleep, nutrition, medication adherence, movement—are stewardship, not self-help. Neglecting known care can become sin by omission (James 4:17).

Radical Acceptance

Accepting reality is not approval of suffering; it is submission to God's sovereignty when change is not immediately given.

Interpersonal Effectiveness

Seeking help becomes faithful when it is timely, bounded, and truthful—not driven by emotional overflow or urgency.

Mindfulness

Observing thoughts and urges without acting honors God's authority over emotion.

Key truth: DBT skills do not replace faith.
They support obedience.

Unity With Differentiation: Roles, Limits, and Order

Romans 12 and 1 Corinthians 12 dismantle the idea that unity requires sameness.

Each member has a role. Each role has limits. Saying no to a role God did not assign is not rejection—it is obedience. Saying yes to one's responsibility, even when costly, is love.

Boundaries are not relational failure.

They are Kingdom order.

They prevent fear from masquerading as peace and emotion from becoming authority.

Speaking the Truth in Love: Skills as Submission[49]

DBT Skill	Spiritual Parallel	Application Example
D – Describe	"Let your conversation be always full of grace." *(Colossians 4:6)*	Speak from observation, not accusation: "I noticed we haven't talked about . . ."

---

[49] The DEAR MAN skill set is part of DBT's Objective Effectiveness, helping individuals communicate needs clearly and respectfully (Linehan 2015).

DBT Skill	Spiritual Parallel	Application Example
E – Express	"Speak the truth in love." *(Ephesians 4:15)*	"I feel hurt when this happens . . ." instead of "You always . . ."
A – Assert	"Say what you mean, mean what you say." *(Matthew 5:37)*	Ask for what you need without guilt or overexplaining.
R – Reinforce	"Encourage one another." *(1 Thessalonians 5:11)*	Thank the person for hearing you, even if it was hard.
GIVE[50] (Gentle, Interested, Validate, Easy manner)	"Be completely humble and gentle." *(Ephesians 4:2)*	Listen with curiosity, validate before correcting.

---

[50] GIVE skills promote relationship effectiveness through gentleness, curiosity, validation, and an easy manner; FAST skills support self-respect by encouraging fairness, value-based boundaries, and truthfulness (Linehan 2015).

DBT Skill	Spiritual Parallel	Application Example
FAST (Fair, no Apologies for Values, Stick to truth, be Truthful)	"Stand firm . . . with the belt of truth." *(Ephesians 6:14)*	Be kind but unwavering when speaking truth.

DBT skills help translate this theology into practice:

- **DEAR MAN** supports *truthful clarity without aggression*

- **GIVE** protects dignity and connection

- **FAST** preserves integrity before God rather than approval from others

Used rightly, these skills do not manage people—they submit communication to Christ's rule.

When Reconciliation Is Slow or Incomplete

Scripture is honest: reconciliation is not always immediate. Sometimes repentance is refused. Sometimes boundaries require distance.

But separation, when it occurs, is always a loss—never a victory.

In the Kingdom, distance is held with grief, prayer, humility, and hope. Unity remains the aim, even when it cannot yet be realized.

It is important to name clearly: faithfulness does not require remaining in unsafe or abusive relationships. Scripture never calls us to submit to harm in the name of unity. In situations where there is ongoing abuse, coercion, or danger, boundaries and distance are not failure—they are obedience. Protecting life, dignity, and safety is not a lack of love; it is alignment with God's heart. Reconciliation requires repentance, truth, and time, and it cannot be forced where those are absent.

Boundaries & Kingdom Order

The Kingdom of God is not chaos or coercion.
It is ordered love under Christ's authority.
Boundaries:

- align us with God first
- clarify responsibility
- protect love from manipulation
- preserve unity without erasing difference

God is not overwhelmed by the complexity of human relationships. He sees motives, wounds, limits, and sin with perfect clarity and perfect love. Our task is not to control outcomes, but to walk faithfully under His rule.

Practice: Preparing to Speak Faithfully

Before your next difficult conversation, pause and ask:

- Am I aligned with God or led by emotion?
- What facts can I state without judgment?
- What responsibility is mine—and what is not?
- What Kingdom objective am I serving?

"Spirit of God, order my love under Your will.
Let my words serve Your Kingdom, not my fear."

Closing Scripture

"I pray that they will all be one . . . so that the world
may believe." (John 17:21)

Unity is not the reward of maturity.
It is the path toward it.
And when truth and love are governed by God's Kingdom,
His presence becomes visible—here, among us.

PART III

The Model:
Jesus, the Divine Integration of the Flesh, Mind, & Spirit

"The Word became flesh and made his dwelling among us. We have seen his glory, the glory of the one and only Son, who came from the Father, full of grace and truth."
—John 1:14

"For God was pleased to have all his fullness dwell in him, and through him to reconcile to himself all things, whether things on earth or things in heaven, by making peace through his blood, shed on the cross."
—Colossians 1:19–20

If Part I revealed the divided mind and Part II invited us to live from the Mind of the Spirit, Part III unveils the fullness of that integration embodied in Christ

Himself—and extended through His Body, the Church. Jesus is not only our example, but is evidence that perfect integration is possible. He is the Word made flesh, where divine wisdom and human experience meet in perfect union. In Him, emotion and reason, compassion and conviction, and heaven and earth converge. His emotions were never repressed; they were redemptive. His reasoning was never detached; it was relational. Every healing, every pause, every word spoken in love flowed from the divine integration of grace and truth.

Yet Jesus did more than model wholeness—He made it possible. Through His sacrifice, He reconciled us to the Father and gathered us into one Body, teaching us to become His living expression on earth. The Church, though imperfect, carries forward His integration: many parts, one Spirit, learning together to think, feel, and love as He does.

This final part explores Jesus as the living embodiment of the Mind-Spirit Bible Practice—and the Church as His ongoing incarnation of that wholeness. In Christ, we discover not only personal healing but a shared communion where grace binds us together—mind, spirit, and flesh—into the family of God.

CHAPTER 7

The Integration: Jesus, the Fullness of the Mind of the Spirit

Who Jesus Is to Me

Before I explore how Jesus embodies perfect integration, I have to start with who He is to me.

Jesus is not just the ultimate case study in spiritual and emotional wholeness—He is my Brother, my Friend, and my Lord. He is both the most human person I know and the most Divine Presence I've ever encountered. His life isn't a theory I admire; it's a relationship that keeps pursuing me.

When I open Scripture, I don't just see lessons about balance or wisdom; I hear the voice of someone who has walked every contradiction I wrestle with. He knows what it's like to feel misunderstood, tired, tempted, and still choose love. The same Jesus who healed the bleeding woman and wept at Lazarus's tomb is the One who sits with me in my living room when my mind is loud, and my heart is heavy.

To me, He isn't an abstract example of integration—He's the living bridge between Heaven and my humanity. His words, "Follow Me," are not an order but an invitation. Every time I lose focus, that same voice whispers, "I believe in you. Let Me show you how."

That is what true discipleship is: not imitation from a distance, but intimacy that transforms. It's learning to let His life inform mine until His compassion shapes my emotions, His clarity steadies my thoughts, and His Spirit becomes the rhythm of my breathing.

That's why, before I can study Jesus as the *model* of the Mind of the Spirit, I have to remember that He is also the *embodiment* of it—alive, personal, and present. Understanding how His mind, emotions, and Spirit moved in perfect harmony isn't about analyzing divinity; it's about recognizing the living Person who still invites us into that same wholeness today.

The Mind of the Spirit Made Flesh

If the previous chapters were glimpses of how the Spirit renews our inner world, this chapter is about how we integrate the Spirit in our physical world. Jesus is not an abstract model of holiness; He is a real, living portrait of emotional, mental, and spiritual integration in human form.

Everywhere Jesus went, you could see balance: feeling

without frenzy, reasoning without rigidity, obedience without fear, compassion without compromise. He lived in perfect communion—the Mind of the Spirit embodied.

From a neuroscientific standpoint, integration occurs when the brain's emotional centers (the limbic system) and rational centers (the prefrontal cortex) communicate effectively through the corpus callosum and vagus nerve pathways. When emotion and reason are in alignment, the nervous system experiences coherence, allowing the body to rest, respond, and relate with empathy. Modern research calls this *neural integration*[51] (Siegel 2012), a state associated with resilience and peace. Theologically, the incarnation of Christ reveals this same reality on a divine level: perfect integration of divinity and humanity—spirit and flesh in absolute coherence. As theologian N.T. Wright (2012) observes, "In Jesus, the life of God and the life of man have become one and the same." The embodied Christ is not only our Redeemer but the truest model of integrated mind, spirit, and body (Siegel 2012).

His mind was never divided between flesh and Spirit, fear and faith. Every response flowed from awareness of the Father's presence. As we see in the book of John, "The Son can do nothing by Himself; He can do only what He sees His Father doing" (5:19).

---

[51] Neural integration refers to the coordination of emotional, cognitive, and physiological processes across brain regions, producing coherence, resilience, and relational attunement (Siegel 2012).

The formation process of Jesus—the way He matured emotionally, mentally, and spiritually—reflects the very integration DBT describes as Wise Mind.[52] Luke 2:52 tells us that "Jesus grew in wisdom and stature, and in favor with God and man." This isn't just moral growth—it's developmental wholeness. He grew cognitively, relationally, and spiritually in perfect alignment. Where DBT teaches mindfulness, Jesus embodied continual awareness[53] of the Father's presence. Where DBT invites us to balance logic and emotion, Jesus lived as truth and compassion in perfect union. His entire formation was integration in motion—the living expression of divine emotional regulation and spiritual maturity.

In the Wilderness—The Mind of the Spirit in Temptation

Each stage of Jesus's ministry mirrors the core competencies of DBT. In the wilderness, He models distress tolerance. In the garden, He practices radical acceptance. On the road, He lives out emotion regulation. And among people, He

---

[52] DBT identifies Wise Mind as the integrated state where logic and emotion function harmoniously, creating clarity, grounded action, and balanced decision-making (Linehan 2015).

[53] Mindfulness in DBT emphasizes sustained present-moment awareness without judgment, enhancing emotional balance and behavioral regulation (Linehan 2015; Bishop et al. 2004).

demonstrates interpersonal effectiveness. His life was not merely holy—it was psychologically whole.

When the Spirit led Jesus into the wilderness, He entered a testing ground familiar to every human soul. Hungry, alone, and exhausted, He faced the same internal conflict we all face:

- The Mind of the Flesh whispered, *"You're starving—turn these stones to bread."*

- The Mind of the World reasoned, *"If You are the Son of God, prove it."*

- But the Mind of the Spirit answered, *"It is written:*[54] *Man shall not live on bread alone"* (Matthew 4:4 ESV).

Where Adam, the first human being, fell to appetite, Jesus, the "Son of Man," stayed aligned with God's Spirit. Jesus did not react out of hunger or pride; He responded out of communion with God.

Every temptation was an invitation to disconnect—to grasp, control, or self-soothe outside of the Father's will. But He remained[55] centered in truth. He showed us that spiritual

---

[54] Distress Tolerance teaches skillful endurance of emotional pain through acceptance, grounding, and non-reactivity rather than impulsive relief-seeking (Linehan 2015).

[55] Wise Mind reflects regulated emotional experience combined with

power is not found in escaping distress but in abiding in God through it.

"It is written . . ." became His distress-tolerance mantra—Scripture as self-soothing, faith as focus, obedience as peace.

In the Garden—Distress Tolerance Perfected

In the Garden of Gethsemane, Jesus carried the weight of human anguish to its limit. He did not hide His pain behind spiritual platitudes. He named it:[56] "My soul is overwhelmed with sorrow to the point of death" (Matthew 26:38).

This is emotional honesty at its purest. He asked His friends to stay near, fell to the ground, and prayed until His sweat became blood. Yet even there, His prayer ended in surrender: ". . . not my will, but yours be done" (Luke 22:42).

That single sentence is Radical Acceptance incarnate.[57] He acknowledged what was unbearable and accepted it

---

clear reasoning, especially critical under distressing or triggering circumstances (Linehan 2015).

[56] Identifying and naming emotions is an Emotion Regulation technique shown to reduce emotional intensity and increase cognitive clarity (Siegel 2012; Linehan 2015).

[57] Radical Acceptance involves fully acknowledging reality—including pain—without resistance, turning toward values-based willingness rather than avoidance or denial (Linehan 2015; Hayes et al. 1999).

without resentment. He neither numbed nor despaired; He stayed present.

Where we panic and reach for false comfort, Jesus prayed until peace returned. Where we avoid, He endured. Where we fracture, He fused human weakness with divine willingness.

This is the highest form of Distress Tolerance—enduring suffering without self-destruction, and finding holiness in the hurt.

Personal Reflection—Sitting in My Own Gethsemane

I often think back to the cliffs in Pacifica—the place where I screamed prayers into the wind, begging God to let me live. The ocean was violent that day, crashing against the rocks like it could feel my panic. My body trembled as I asked, *"Please, don't let this be the end of my story."* I wasn't ready to die; I wasn't ready to lose the life I knew at age 23 and the future I had hoped for.

At that moment, I felt closer to Jesus in Gethsemane than ever before. At that moment, Jesus was no longer a character or story in a book; I could see Him, feel Him, and it felt as if I could touch Him. His words, "My Father, if it is possible, let this cup pass from me," (Matthew 26:39 ESV) stopped being scripture on a page and became oxygen in my lungs. I was begging God for my life, just like Jesus did. For the first time, I understood that He wasn't just fulfilling prophecy—He was fully feeling what it means to be human: terrified, trembling, and choosing obedience anyway.

That realization grounded me; it opened my mind to experiencing scripture not just as a "nice thought" or "interesting concept," but it made scripture human and real. This real human being, Jesus Christ, who was also God, was dying. The idea that a Deity would *want* to experience human suffering so that He could empathize with me, so that I would never have to suffer alone, changed the way I see pain. Jesus didn't numb, avoid, or control His anguish; He practiced the purest form of what DBT calls Radical Acceptance—acknowledging unbearable reality while remaining surrendered to love. He didn't flee distress; He tolerated it with faith. He didn't suppress emotion; He let it move through Him until it became prayer.

As I sat on that cliff, breathing through tears, I realized that the same Mind of the Spirit that steadied Jesus in Gethsemane was steadying me. DBT gives me the language—*observe, name, accept, breathe*—but Jesus gave me the revelation: acceptance is not resignation; it's relationship. It's the holy pause between "take this cup" and "not my will but Yours."

In that space, I found both therapy and theology meeting in the same heartbeat. My suffering became communion. My trembling became prayer. And peace—fragile but real—entered like a whisper, saying, "I know this pain. I've carried it too." Jesus wasn't just empathizing with me anymore; I was learning to empathize with Him.

And just as the Father strengthened Jesus after the

garden, I found strength too—enough to rise from the cliffs of Pacifica and keep walking. What came next was the slow work of emotional regulation: learning to let that same peace guide my steps.

On the Road—Emotional Regulation in Motion

Jesus felt everything.

He wept at Lazarus's tomb—showing us that tears are spiritual, not shameful. He rejoiced in the Spirit when His disciples grasped truth. He grew angry when the temple was exploited—anger purified by love of justice, not fueled by ego. He lamented over Jerusalem, grieving those who rejected truth and grace.

Every emotion found its rightful rhythm in Him.[58] Nothing was suppressed; nothing was exaggerated. His emotional life was perfectly regulated because His identity was perfectly secure.

Peace ruled His reactions. Where we spiral between Emotion Mind and Reason Mind, Jesus remained in Wise Mind—the Mind of the Spirit. He felt deeply and still acted wisely. As Scripture says, "You will keep in perfect peace those whose minds are steadfast, because they trust in You" (Isaiah 26:3).

---

[58] Emotion Regulation skills help individuals modulate emotional responses by cultivating identity stability, reducing vulnerability factors, and increasing grounded awareness (Linehan 2015).

Among People—Interpersonal Effectiveness Embodied

Jesus's relationships reveal the divine art of speaking the truth in love. He spoke boldly to the self-righteous, yet gently to the broken. He set boundaries without bitterness and showed compassion without compromise. When I practice truth in love with the people closest to me, I often think of these moments—Jesus restoring Peter, Jesus seeing the woman no one else saw.

To the woman caught in adultery, He said: "Neither do I condemn you. Go now and leave your life of sin" (John 8:11*). Grace and truth, held in one breath.

To Peter, who denied Him, He offered restoration instead of resentment: "Do you love Me? . . . Feed My sheep" (John 21:17).

To Judas, who betrayed Him, He offered friendship and love until the end.

Every conversation was balanced—objective, relational, and self-respecting.

He embodied every DBT skill we've learned:[59]

- Describe: He stated facts without accusation.

- Express: He shared emotion without manipulation.

---

[59] DBT's Interpersonal Effectiveness skills—DEAR MAN, GIVE, FAST—support clear communication, relational attunement, and self-respect during interpersonal exchanges (Linehan 2015).

- Assert: He spoke His needs clearly.
- Reinforce: He offered hope for transformation.
- Validate: He saw people before correcting them.

His communication was never about control; it was about *connection*. He showed us that spiritual maturity is relational maturity.

At the Cross—Full Integration

On the cross, every concept of this book meets its fulfillment.[60]

- Distress Tolerance: He endured unimaginable pain without self-pity.

- Emotion Regulation: He expressed sorrow, not rage—"My God, my God, why have You forsaken Me?" (Matthew 27:46 ESV)—but stayed conscious of God's presence.

- Interpersonal Effectiveness: He extended forgiveness even to His killers—"Father, forgive them . . ." (Luke 23:34 ESV).

- Mind of the Spirit: He remained aligned—"Father, into Your hands I commit My Spirit!" (Luke 23:46 ESV)

---

[60] Crisis survival skills help individuals endure overwhelming situations without resorting to harmful or impulsive actions—often involving grounding, acceptance, and value-aligned behavior (Linehan 2015).

In Jesus, humanity and divinity meet, perfectly integrated. His final breath tore the veil between God and man, proving that emotional and spiritual alignment is not a distant ideal—it is the gift Jesus bought for us with His blood.

As John 7:38 says, "Whoever believes in Me, rivers of living water will flow from within them." That living water is the Spirit who now dwells in us—the same Spirit that sustained Jesus through wilderness, garden, and cross.

Resurrection—The Renewal of All Things

Three days later, this integration became power. Resurrection is the ultimate proof that endurance in the Spirit is never wasted. Where despair ends for the world, new life begins in God.

In DBT language, resurrection is the transformation stage—when integration produces vitality.

In spiritual language, it is being made holy—the soul made whole through suffering. Revelation 21:5 says, "Behold, I am making all things new."

The same Spirit who raised Jesus from the dead is the One who raises our emotional, relational, and spiritual life from fragmentation to freedom.

Living the Integration—Our Invitation

To live "in Christ" is to participate in His integration. The same Spirit that ordered His thoughts and emotions now teaches us the slow, sanctifying work of regulation and alignment. DBT calls this the practice of Wise Mind—a steady return to center.[61] Scripture calls it *abiding in the Vine* (John 15:1-8). Both describe a life where awareness becomes repentance, self-control becomes fruit, and emotional honesty becomes communion with God and others.

Every skill of DBT becomes, in Christ, a form of spiritual formation:

- **Mindfulness** becomes *abiding* in God (John 15:4–5).

- **Radical Acceptance** becomes *surrender* ("Not my will, but Yours be done").

- **Emotion Regulation** becomes "peace that surpasses understanding" (Philippians 4:7).

- **Interpersonal Effectiveness** becomes *truth in love* (Ephesians 4:15).

These practices, when submitted to the Spirit, are not self-help—they are participation in divine life.

To live from the Mind of the Spirit is to allow our neurobiology, psychology, and spirituality to be rewired by grace. The Spirit does not erase our humanity; He integrates it.

---

[61] Wise Mind is cultivated not through perfection but through continual returning to awareness, balance, and aligned action when the mind becomes dysregulated (Linehan 2015).

Every part of us—body, emotion, thought, and spirit—can be redeemed into alignment with God's heart.

Jesus doesn't just show us how to live this integration; He lives this integration *through* us. The Spirit that ruled His heart now inhabits ours. "And we all . . . are being transformed into His image with ever-increasing glory . . ." (2 Corinthians 3:18).

The practices of the Mind-Spirit Bible Practice—mindfulness, radical acceptance, repentance, truth in love—are not self-help habits; they are ways of staying in union with Him.

Every wilderness becomes a place of revelation.
Every emotion becomes a doorway to intimacy.
Every conversation becomes an altar of reconciliation.
Every surrender becomes participation in His divine life.

Reflection and Practice

Scripture Meditation

"Whoever claims to live in Him must live as Jesus did" (1 John 2:6).

Practice of Integration

1. Recall the four paths: Mind of the Spirit, Distress Tolerance, Emotion Regulation, Interpersonal Effectiveness.

2. Identify one area where you still feel divided or disconnected.

3. Ask: *How did Jesus live this?*

4. Pray: *God, help me align my mind and heart with Yours.*

5. Act: Take one small step in imitation—breathe, forgive, speak truth, or wait in trust.

Prayer

"God, You gave Jesus, the perfect integration of humanity and divinity.

Teach me to think as He thought, to feel as He felt, to love as He loved.

When I am distressed, anchor me in surrender.

When emotion floods, rule my heart with peace.

When relationships strain, guide my tongue with truth and grace.

Let Your living water flow through me until my life, too, becomes communion with You. Amen."

Walking With Him Still

When I look back on my own story, I realize the goal has never been perfect balance—it's been deeper friendship. The same Jesus who walked through the wilderness, garden, and cross now walks with me through grocery aisles, late-night worries, and small acts of forgiveness.

He still whispers the same words He spoke in Galilee: "Follow Me." Only now, I hear them not as a demand for perfection, but as an invitation into presence.

Every time I pause to breathe before reacting, every time I forgive, every time I surrender what I cannot control—I feel Him there, smiling, saying, "You're learning. I believe in you."

The integration I once studied has become my best friend. Jesus is not just the map; He is the walking partner who makes this life's journey worth living.

Closing Thought

Jesus is not merely the example of wholeness; He is its source. In Him, the wilderness becomes worship, emotion becomes empathy, truth becomes love, and suffering becomes resurrection.

To live in the Mind of the Spirit is to live in Christ Himself—steady, surrendered, honest, and whole. As Philippians says, "Let this mind be in you, which was also in Christ Jesus" (2:5 KJV).

This is the culmination of Mind-Spirit Bible Practice: not escaping our humanity, but redeeming it—until our hearts, like His, become the dwelling place of perfect peace.

The story of Jesus is the story of integration made visible—the divine and the human held together in unbroken love. In Him, we glimpse the final harmony of creation: every neuron, every emotion, every act of compassion synchronized under divine peace. When Paul writes, "In Him all things hold together" (Colossians 1:17), it includes us, our minds and bodies, our sorrows and strengths. Christ is not merely the healer of fragmentation; He is the architecture of wholeness itself. To follow Him is to live as integrated beings—mind renewed, spirit awakened, and body participating in the ongoing incarnation of grace.

CHAPTER 8

The Body of Christ:
The Banquet of Adoption

"In love He predestined us for adoption to sonship through Jesus Christ, in accordance with His pleasure and will"

—Ephesians 1:4–5

"Above all, clothe yourselves with love, which binds us all together in perfect unity."

—Colossians 3:14

The Adoptive Heart of God

One morning in prayer, I was missing my foster sons, who had recently been reunified with their biological family. The grief of losing them hurt so deeply that it was hard to breathe. I whispered through tears, "I'd do anything to get them back—just to follow them around, watch them grow, hold them again." And then I heard the Spirit whisper, "That's how I feel about you."

In that moment, I understood, not just intellectually but emotionally, what God's adoptive love feels like—the ache, the longing, the fierce desire to reconcile what's lost. God could have filled creation with flawless, spiritually "biological" children, but He chose instead to become a Father through adoption—fully knowing the heartbreak and beauty it would require. It wasn't His last resort; adoption was His first choice for how God wanted to build His family. Ephesians says, "God decided in advance to adopt us into His own family by bringing us to Himself through Jesus Christ" (1:5 NLT). He knew we would come with trauma, mistrust, culture, and history. And still He said, "I want you."

But adoption is risky and costly. Someone has to take the risk and stand in the gap. That is what Jesus did. He became the bridge between heaven and humanity—the mediator who bore our estrangement so we could come home. By His sacrifice, we are not just forgiven; we are welcomed. By His wounds, the door of the Father's house swung open. Through His death and resurrection, He signed our adoption papers with His own blood, making us legal heirs of grace.

I recently bought a bigger house, and I hope to foster-adopt one day; yet I still keep a clean room ready for my foster sons, with all their toys and favorite blankets, just in case they ever need it again. I hope one day to be reunited with them, in some capacity, in some way—and whatever condition they are in, I will accept and long to embrace them.

In the same way, God keeps a room ready for every one of us—prepared through the work of Christ—hoping for our return, eager to embrace us no matter our condition. "My Father's house has many rooms . . . I am going to prepare a place for you" (John 14:2).

That is the heart of adoption: to prepare a place, to say, "You still belong here." Jesus is the reason that door will never close.

This is the heart of God's will on earth: not merely the healing of individuals, but the formation of a family. God's Kingdom is not an abstract idea or a distant future—it is His rule made visible through a people learning to live together under His love. The Church, for all its imperfections, is the present expression of that will. It is not the Kingdom in its fullness, but it is the place where the Kingdom is practiced, embodied, and worked out over time. Integration, then, is never complete in isolation. It reaches its fullness only as we learn to belong, to tell the truth, to love, and to mature together in the Body Christ is still forming.

The Banquet of the Father

Jesus told of a great banquet where those first invited refused to come. So the master sent servants to the streets and alleys to gather *everyone*—the broken, the poor, the blind, the lame. That is the gospel: an open invitation to belong.

But in another parable (Matthew 22), a guest arrived without wedding clothes. The story wasn't about exclusion—it was about preparation. The Father invites all to His table and then teaches us how to be dressed for love.

DBT mirrors this wisdom: awareness, acceptance, and regulation are spiritual garments.[62]

We cannot sit at the banquet wearing shame, rage, or self-condemnation; we must let the Spirit re-dress us in compassion, patience, and peace. To *clothe ourselves with love* is to choose Wise Mind—alignment with the Spirit before action.

DBT Skill	Spiritual Garment	Practice
Mindfulness	Awareness of God's presence	Notice what you're emotionally "wearing."
Distress Tolerance	Persevering love	Stay at the table when it's uncomfortable.[63]

---

[62] DBT's Mindfulness practices cultivate nonjudgmental awareness of internal experience and promote emotional and behavioral alignment with values—functioning as foundational "garments" for regulated living (Linehan 2015).

[63] Distress Tolerance skills help individuals remain present during emotional discomfort without resorting to avoidance, impulsivity, or relational withdrawal—strengthening endurance and connection (Linehan 2015).

DBT Skill	Spiritual Garment	Practice
Emotion Regulation	Peace that surpasses understanding	Name the feeling; invite the truth to re-dress it.[64]
Interpersonal Effectiveness	Speaking truth in love	Set boundaries with grace, not guilt.[65]

The Father's banquet is full of messy, beautiful people in process. We are all learning how to wear love well.

When we learn to wear these garments, we stop performing and start participating. We discover that love isn't a feeling to achieve—it's a garment to live in. But even when we wander from the table, the Father's invitation remains open.

This is why the work of the Kingdom unfolds slowly. There are seasons when we are asked simply to remain with God while nothing changes, learning endurance rather than resolution. There are seasons when the primary work

---

[64] Emotion Regulation skills include identifying emotions accurately, reducing vulnerability factors, and replacing unhelpful emotional responses with value-aligned behaviors (Linehan 2015; Siegel 2012).

[65] Interpersonal Effectiveness assists individuals in expressing needs, setting boundaries, and maintaining self-respect while sustaining relational connection—often through DEAR MAN, GIVE, and FAST skills (Linehan 2015).

is inward—tending to the emotions that rise while we wait, learning how to return to God instead of being ruled by fear or reactivity. And there are seasons when faithfulness takes shape between us, as we learn to speak the truth in love, to honor boundaries, and to remain connected without control. None of this work is separate. Together, it is how God forms a people who can carry His presence in the world.

The Return Home

When I think of God's adoptive heart, I see myself in the prodigal son. I've run, doubted, and hidden. I've manipulated, trying to get my way, and strived to earn my worth.

"While he was still a long way off, his father saw him and was filled with compassion . . . he ran to his son, threw his arms around him and kissed him" (Luke 15:20). Yet, just like in the story of the prodigal son, each time I return to the Spirit, back into alignment with God, my Father God runs toward me—arms wide, tears streaming, no lecture, only love.

The robe He places on us is identity. The ring is belonging. It's not just forgiveness; it's reintegration. 1 John 4:17-19 says, "By living in God, love has been brought to its full expression in us . . . Love never brings fear . . . Our love for others is our grateful response to the love God first demonstrated to us" (TPT).

Love is the door home and the robe we wear when we get there.

Adopted by the Church

When I look back over my life, I see how God's adoptive love reached me through His people.

The Church became His nervous system—transmitting His compassion through a woven tapestry of ordinary, faithful lives.

There were families who took me in, who fed me, prayed with me, and never made me feel like a burden. Leaders who listened to my tears, spoke truth with gentleness, and believed in who I could become. Friends who helped me heal after brain surgery, brought meals when I was sick, and reminded me that God still had a purpose for my pain. They didn't fix me—they stayed. They modeled love through consistency, patience, and presence.

Through them, God re-parented me. He taught me that faith is not just what happens in church buildings; it's what happens around kitchen tables, in hospital rooms, and through text messages that say, *"I'm still here."*

But I also know not everyone has experienced the Church this way. Many have felt unseen or hurt by the very people meant to represent God's love. If that's you, I want to gently remind you: the Church is not a perfect institution—it's a living, growing body made up of broken people learning to love like Christ.

Wherever you are, you can begin again.[66] You can be part of God's healing nervous system in the world—by becoming the one who listens, feeds, prays, and stays.

To be adopted into God's family is to be continually re-formed into love. It's learning to sit at the banquet table beside others with different stories, to show up clothed not in self-protection but in compassion: "Therefore, as God's chosen people, holy and dearly loved, clothe yourselves with compassion, kindness, humility, gentleness, and patience. And over all these virtues, put on love, which binds them all together in perfect unity" (Colossians 3:12–14).

These people didn't just talk about God's love—they embodied it. Through them, God led me "with cords of human kindness, with ties of love" (Hosea 11:4). Yet the invitation remains for all of us: to keep becoming that embodiment for someone else. The Church is not a place you attend; it's a life you participate in—one act of love at a time.

Their lives taught me DBT skills before I had names for them: mindful presence, distress tolerance, emotion regulation, and interpersonal effectiveness—all wrapped in grace.

They showed me how to stay at the table, how to calm through connection, how to speak truth without shame.

------

[66] Validation—accurately acknowledging another's internal experience—is central to DBT relational repair, improving connection, reducing conflict, and strengthening trust (Linehan 2015; Lynch 2018).

Love as the Culture of Heaven

DBT taught me to integrate emotion and reason; Christ taught me to integrate heaven and earth. In Him, everything fragmented finds alignment. He is the Head of the Body; in Him we hold together.

The early Church modeled this integration: "They sold property and possessions to give to anyone who had need . . . praising God and enjoying the favor of all the people" (Acts 2:45-47).

Integration is not solitary but communal. We heal in households, in conversations, in bread-breaking moments where grace gets tangible. Every act of patience and presence becomes a thread in the garment of love that binds us together in Christ.

1 John expands on this type of love:

Delightfully loved ones, if He loved us with such tremendous love, then "loving one another" should be our way of life! . . . if we love one another, God makes His permanent home in us . . . He has given us His Spirit within us so that we can have the assurance that He lives in us and we live in Him. (4:11-13 TPT)

When we love one another, the invisible God becomes visible through us. This is both theology and therapy—the divine nervous system regulating the world through connection. DBT calls it *co-regulation;* Scripture calls it *communion.*[67]

We are all adoptees learning the culture of our new home—the culture of heaven. Love is the language; grace is the accent. Fear has no citizenship here. It says later in 1 John, "Love never brings fear . . . love's perfection drives the fear of punishment far from our hearts" (4:18 TPT*).*

Adoption doesn't erase difference; it redeems it. In God's family, each of us arrives with our own story, culture, and coping style. Some are expressive, others reserved; some come from scarcity, others from excess. But we're learning to live under one roof—the Father's.

DBT calls this *walking the middle path*—holding both acceptance and change at once.[68] The Body of Christ lives in that tension too: we accept one another as we are, yet we also call one another to transformation. Grace doesn't mean passivity; it means staying in relationship long enough for the Spirit to do His work. Just as families learn to balance validation and accountability, the Church learns to love with truth and tenderness at the same time.

---

[67] Co-regulation refers to the process through which nervous systems stabilize through connection with others; mindfulness-based therapies highlight interpersonal attunement as a key mechanism for emotional regulation (Siegel 2012; Linehan 2015).

[68] Walking the Middle Path is a DBT skill that balances acceptance and change, helping individuals navigate family differences, emotional extremes, and relational tension with flexibility (Linehan 2015).

Discipleship means being re-parented by grace—learning to love like our new family loves. It isn't always easy. We trigger each other. We misunderstand. But we stay, pray, forgive, and begin again. We learn the rhythms of our new home until they become second nature.

That is integration: the Spirit teaching our bodies and souls to rest in belonging.

Pause & Practice—Wearing the Clothes of Love

- **Observe:** What "clothes" are you wearing emotionally today[69]—fear, pride, resentment, or compassion?

- **Describe:** Ask God, "What do You want me to put on instead?"

- **Participate:** Practice one DBT skill that helps you embody love[70]—mindful breathing, gentle tone, validating someone's emotion, speaking truth in love.

---

[69] Mindfulness of current emotion is a DBT strategy that encourages observing and describing emotional states without judgment, increasing regulation and relational presence (Linehan 2015).

[70] DBT's interpersonal skills teach individuals how to communicate with gentleness, fairness, emotional attunement, and integrity—enabling "embodied" expressions of love and connection (Linehan 2015).

- **Affirm:** "Father, thank You for adopting me into Your family. Teach me to wear Your love like Jesus did."

The Church is God's banquet—an imperfect table filled with adopted children still learning how to eat together. We are different, but we belong. We are wounded, but we are wanted. We are being clothed, daily, in love. And love—the language of heaven—keeps teaching us how to stay at the table.

The Church is not a finished house; it is a family still learning how to live together. We will misunderstand one another. We will need truth to keep purifying us and love to keep binding us. And Jesus—the One who holds all things together—will remain faithful to His work in us until the day unity is complete.

Jesus is not only the One who holds all things together; He is the Head of the Church, from whom the whole Body grows, finds its order, and is held in unity until the day His work in us is complete (Colossians 1:17–18; Ephesians 1:22–23).

This is where the journey leads—not to perfection, but to participation. We are sent back into ordinary life as adopted children learning the culture of our Father's house: staying when it would be easier to leave, speaking truth when silence feels safer, choosing love when fear tempts us to withdraw. God's will is not accomplished all at once, but slowly, faithfully, through a people willing to keep showing up.

Until the day we see Him face to face, this is our calling: to live as citizens of the Kingdom now, trusting that what is incomplete will be made whole, and that even our imperfect love is being gathered into something eternal.

This is now yours to live—not perfectly, but faithfully. Not in isolation, but in the Body God has placed you in. You will stumble, misunderstand, and begin again. And still, Christ remains the Head who holds you, the Church that carries you, and the Kingdom that is growing through your ordinary obedience. Faithfulness does not require mastery—only presence, truth, and love practiced over time. As you leave these pages, you do not leave the work behind. You carry it into real relationships, real communities, and real moments where God's will is quietly being done on earth, through you.

A Reflection Before You Go

If you've made it this far, thank you. You've just walked through the wilderness, garden, and cross with me—and, I hope, with Jesus too. Writing this book has not been an academic project for me; it has been a survival story, a healing journey, and a prayer in motion.

I didn't write *The Mind-Spirit Bible Practice* because I had all the answers. I wrote it because I *needed* it. I needed a framework that could hold what I was learning in therapy, what I was reading in my morning devotionals, and what I was experiencing in the tension between my human reality and the supernatural presence of God. This process has not only been thought-provoking—it has been profoundly healing. I will keep reading these pages myself, again and again, as reminders of the relationship that continually makes me whole and integrated.

I began this book searching for balance. I wanted peace, regulation, and a way to hold my faith and my emotions without feeling like one disqualified the other. What I found instead was a relationship—a God who does not merely teach integration but *embodies it.*

Jesus never promised that walking with Him would mean an even, regulated life. But He did promise His presence. He promised a Helper—the same Spirit who hovered over the waters of creation and now hovers over our chaos, bringing order from within.

My prayer is that as you continue this journey, you won't just practice these skills—you'll practice *companionship.* You'll notice Jesus beside you in the smallest moments: in your breath before a hard conversation, in your pause before a reaction, in your surrender when control slips through your fingers.

If anything in these pages has met you where you are, let it remind you: wholeness isn't a destination. It's the slow, holy friendship that forms when we let Jesus walk with us— day after day, emotion by emotion, until His peace becomes our natural rhythm.

Along this journey, God also revealed His presence through His people—the Church. They became His hands, His words, His patience, and His provision when I needed it most. Every ride to church, every meal shared, every prayer whispered over me was a thread in the tapestry of healing. The Body of Christ—imperfect, human, and holy—has been the living classroom where I learned what grace looks like in motion. My hope is that as you walk forward, you'll not only meet Jesus in solitude but also rediscover Him in community—the kind that listens, prays, stays, and loves you back into life.

Thank you for letting me share my story. May the same Spirit that steadied Jesus in Gethsemane steady you now—until every wilderness becomes revelation, and every moment becomes communion.

With love and gratitude,
—Nicole Doña

The Practice Continues

Sometimes, I live from the Mind of the Spirit—breathing truth, listening to God's Spirit. Other days, I forget everything I've written in this book. I fall back into my old patterns: reacting from fear, reasoning without listening, trying to control what I was never meant to.

But I've learned this: every time I lose my way, Jesus is still there—patient, steady, unshaken.

The Spirit never stops whispering,

"I'm still here. Just listen."

That whisper is the invitation I want to leave with you.

Because this practice—this Mind-Spirit Bible Practice—is not about getting it right; it's about *returning*. It's about learning to pause before reacting, to breathe before speaking, to listen before fixing. It's about noticing when you've slipped into the mind of the flesh or the mind of the world, and then gently, humbly, coming back to the Mind of the

Spirit—where peace surpasses understanding and grace meets you exactly where you are.

You don't have to master this. You just have to *begin.* Begin again tomorrow if you lose it tonight. Begin again in the car, or in the kitchen, or while crying on the bathroom floor. Because every breath is another chance to begin with God.

My hope is that you'll let this practice become yours— that you'll learn to sit with Jesus in your wilderness, to let the Spirit steady your heart in the storm, and to find your words again in love, not fear.

May you remember that Jesus isn't waiting at the finish line—He's walking with you in the practice. He is the peace you're practicing toward.

So don't give up when it feels slow. Don't stop when you slip. Keep showing up to the Presence that never leaves.

And one day, you'll look back and realize—you didn't just study the Mind of the Spirit.

You lived it.

You became it.

You walked with Him, and He walked with you—every step of the way.

Acknowledgments

This book was not written alone. It was held, shaped, and sustained by a community of people who prayed with me, walked with me through joy and suffering, and believed in the vision of the Mind–Spirit Bible Practice long before it was fully formed. Each of you offered your presence, wisdom, or love at a moment when I needed it most. I am forever grateful.

Becky & Zach Mariscal
Bobbi & Mark Higuera
Cynthia Beach
Dany & Lina Mendez
Denise Crowl
Doris & Gabriel Lacayo
Eddie & Michelle Marquez
Esmond Chia & Tessa Kwan
Lauren Marquez
Miguel & Charvette Rojas
Natasha Crawford

Nathan & Audrey Spaun
Poppy Anderson
Ralph & Yumiko Eisley
Rebekah & Sandor Manuel
Ruth Corliss
Shane & Wendy Ballew
Shayla Murphy
Shondricka Burrell
Starr Herron
Wendi & Chuck Anderson

You are the ones who helped me believe that healing is possible, that love is stronger than fear, and that God is still writing a beautiful story through His people. This book is as much yours as it is mine.

Appendix: Integrating DBT With Spiritual Formation

The Mind–Spirit Bible Practice is built on a simple truth:

our emotional life and our spiritual life were never meant to be separate.

Throughout this book, you've encountered concepts and skills from **Dialectical Behavior Therapy (DBT)**—an evidence-based framework created by Dr. Marsha Linehan to help people regulate emotions, build resilience, improve relationships, and develop healthy coping strategies.

Rather than offering DBT as a clinical tool, this book uses it as a **lens of emotional wisdom**, pairing it with Scripture to illuminate how:

- the *Mind of the Spirit* integrates what emotion and logic often tear apart,

- the *Way of Jesus* provides the ultimate model of emotional and relational wholeness,

- and the *Body of Christ* becomes a living, co-regulating nervous system of love.

This Appendix is designed to help you:

- understand each DBT concept you encountered,
- revisit skills that resonated with you,
- deepen your emotional-spiritual practice,
- and find specific chapters where each concept appears.

Whether you're a mental-health professional, ministry leader, or a person simply seeking emotional and spiritual transformation, this glossary and index will help you move from insight to integration—from theory into embodied practice.

APPENDIX A

How This Book Relates to Therapy

Many readers encounter this book while already engaged in therapy, while others may be considering it, and some may be uncertain or cautious due to past experiences. This appendix is offered to clarify how *The Mind–Spirit Bible Practice* is meant to relate to therapeutic work.

This Book Is Not Therapy

This book does not provide diagnoses, treatment plans, or clinical instruction. It does not replace psychotherapy, psychiatric care, or crisis support. Rather, it reflects one person's experience of integrating psychological tools with Christian spiritual formation.

This Book May Complement Therapy

For readers who are in therapy, the practices in this book may:

- Provide spiritual language for experiences already being explored clinically

- Support emotional awareness, distress tolerance, and values-aligned living

- Help integrate faith into therapeutic work where that dimension has felt absent or fragmented

Many readers may find it helpful to discuss insights from this book with a therapist, pastor, or spiritual director, especially when strong emotions or memories arise.

Psychological Concepts Are Used as Bridges, Not Authority

Where concepts from Dialectical Behavior Therapy (DBT) and related approaches appear, they are used descriptively and metaphorically—as bridges between emotional experience and spiritual practice. These frameworks help name patterns many people already live with, but they are not presented as exhaustive explanations of the human person.

Theological reflection and Scripture remain the central interpretive lens of this book.

When Therapy Is Especially Important

Readers experiencing active trauma symptoms, suicidal thoughts, severe emotional distress, or functional impairment are strongly encouraged to seek professional care. Doing so is not a lack of faith; it is an act of stewardship, humility, and wisdom.

Christian faith has always affirmed the value of embodied care, community support, and shared burden-bearing. Therapy can be one of the ways God provides that care.

A Final Word on Integration

Integration, as described in this book, is not about blending faith and psychology into a single system. It is about **learning to live as a whole person**—mind, body, and spirit—under the loving authority of God.

Therapy can help clear space. Spiritual practice can help us remain present. Neither replaces the other, and both can serve the work of healing when held with humility, discernment, and grace.

DBT + Scripture Crosswalk Charts

A Bridge Between Psychological Skill and Spiritual Formation

These charts help readers see that the emotional skills taught in DBT echo and illuminate truths God has already woven into Scripture. Use it to deepen reflection, teaching, and spiritual practice.

MIND STATES

DBT Concept	Description	Scripture Parallel	Biblical Insight
Emotion Mind	Emotion drives behavior; impulsivity, overwhelm.	Psalm 42; Psalm 55	The psalmists often describe emotional floods and impulses without shame.
Reason Mind	Logic without emotion; detachment, overthinking.	Proverbs 3:5–7	Relying only on our own understanding leads to disconnection and pride.

DBT Concept	Description	Scripture Parallel	Biblical Insight
Wise Mind	Integration of emotion + reason; inner wisdom.	Isaiah 30:21; John 14:26; Romans 8:6	The Spirit guides, integrates, and brings clarity beyond logic or emotion.

MINDFULNESS SKILLS

DBT Skill	Description	Scripture Parallel	Biblical Insight
Observe	Notice internal experience without reacting.	Psalm 46:10	"Be still and know . . ."—awareness before action.
Describe	Label thoughts/emotions accurately.	Psalm 62:8	Pour out your heart; name what is true.

DBT Skill	Description	Scripture Parallel	Biblical Insight
Participate	Enter the moment fully.	Colossians 3:17	Whatever you do, do it wholeheartedly in God's presence.
Non-judg-mentally	Observe without condemning yourself.	Romans 8:1	No condemnation—honest awareness without shame.
One-Mind-fully	Focus on one thing at a time.	Matthew 6:22–24	A "single eye" brings clarity and alignment.
Effectively	Act based on what works, not what feels good.	1 Corinthians 10:23	"Not everything is beneficial"—choose what leads to life.

DISTRESS TOLERANCE

DBT Skill	Description	Scripture Parallel	Biblical Insight
Radical Acceptance	Accepting reality without resistance.	Luke 22:42	Jesus's Gethsemane prayer: "Not My will . . ."
Turning the Mind	Re-committing to acceptance repeatedly.	Psalm 131:2	"I have calmed and quieted my soul."
Willingness vs. Willfulness	Yielding vs. resisting reality.	Jonah 1–4	Jonah's willfulness vs. God's invitation to willingness.
Self-Soothing	Calming through the five senses.	1 Kings 19:5–13	God soothes Elijah with rest, food, whisper.

DBT Skill	Description	Scripture Parallel	Biblical Insight
IMPROVE the Moment	Micro-practices to create relief.	Philippians 4:6–8	Prayer, gratitude, meditation, choosing what is good.
Crisis Survival	Endure pain without making it worse.	Psalm 23; Daniel 3	Walking with God *in* the fire, not around it.

EMOTION REGULATION

DBT Skill	Description	Scripture Parallel	Biblical Insight
Understanding Emotions	Emotions communicate needs/values.	Ephesians 4:26	"Be angry, but sin not"—emotion itself is not sin.
Labeling Emotions	Reduces emotional intensity.	Psalm 38; Psalm 13	Biblical leaders name sadness, fear, rage, despair.

DBT Skill	Description	Scripture Parallel	Biblical Insight
Opposite Action	Doing the opposite of destructive impulses.	Romans 12:21	Overcome evil with good; action transforms emotion.
Checking the Facts	Testing whether emotions fit reality.	2 Corinthians 10:5	Taking thoughts captive; evaluating what is true.
ABC PLEASE	Reducing vulnerability to emotional overwhelm.	1 Kings 19	Elijah's burn-out story: sleep, food, rest—before mission.
Build Mastery	Daily practices that build competence.	Proverbs 6:6–8	Discipline, diligence, small steps produce strength.

DBT Skill	Description	Scripture Parallel	Biblical Insight
Cope Ahead	Preparing for emotionally difficult situations.	Matthew 26:36–46	Jesus prepares Himself in Gethsemane before the cross.

INTERPERSONAL EFFECTIVENESS

DBT Skill	Description	Scripture Parallel	Biblical Insight
DEAR MAN	Clear, assertive communication.	Matthew 18:15	Go directly, speak clearly, address issues lovingly.
GIVE	Gentle, validating communication.	Colossians 4:6	Speech full of grace, seasoned with salt.
FAST	Maintaining self-respect.	Proverbs 4:23	Guard your heart—honor your values.

DBT Skill	Description	Scripture Parallel	Biblical Insight
Validation	Acknowledging another's internal world.	Romans 12:15	"Weep with those who weep."
Boundary-Setting	Protecting integrity + connection.	Mark 1:35–38	Jesus sets boundaries to pray, rest, and stay aligned.
Walking the Middle Path	Holding both acceptance and change.	John 1:14	Jesus is "full of grace *and* truth."
Co-regulation	Calming through connection.	Galatians 6:2	Bear one another's burdens; shared nervous systems.

INTEGRATION & IDENTITY

Concept	Description	Scripture Parallel	Biblical Insight
Integration	Aligning emotion, thought, behavior, and spirit.	Colossians 1:17	"In Him all things hold together."
Belonging / Adoption	Rooted identity reduces emotional chaos.	Ephesians 1:5	Adoption brings emotional grounding and security.
Embodied Love	Skillful action aligned with compassion.	1 John 4; John 13	Love made visible through behavior.

MASTER DBT GLOSSARY

MIND STATES

Emotion Mind

A state where emotions dominate thinking and behavior. Decisions are driven by feelings—sometimes impulsively, sometimes intensely—making it hard to see clearly.

Reason Mind

A state grounded in logic, analysis, problem-solving, and facts—often helpful, but can disconnect us from emotional truth and relational presence.

Wise Mind

The integration of Emotion Mind and Reason Mind. A grounded, intuitive, Spirit-aligned awareness that holds emotion and truth together. DBT's closest parallel to the biblical "Mind of the Spirit."

MINDFULNESS SKILLS

Observe

Noticing internal or external experience without trying to change it. Watching thoughts, emotions, and sensations like clouds moving across the sky.

Describe

Putting words to your experience ("My chest feels tight," "I'm noticing sadness"). Naming reduces overwhelm and creates emotional separation.

Participate

Entering the present moment fully—heart, mind, and body—rather than splitting off, numbing out, or overthinking.

Non-judgmentally

Letting go of labels like "good," "bad," "weak," or "too much." Viewing experience with compassion and curiosity.

One-Mindfully

Focusing on one thing at a time—a thought, task, breath, prayer—rather than multitasking or mentally spiraling.

Effectively

Acting in ways that work—not to win, be right, or avoid discomfort, but to align with your values and produce peace.

DISTRESS TOLERANCE SKILLS

Radical Acceptance

Fully acknowledging reality as it is—not approving of it, not resigning to it—but surrendering resistance so suffering decreases.

Turning the Mind

Re-committing to acceptance each time the mind resists. A spiritual parallel to repeatedly returning to God.

Willingness vs. Willfulness

Willingness: cooperating with reality and God's guidance.

Willfulness: resisting, shutting down, refusing, or demanding control.

Self-Soothing

Using the five senses (touch, smell, sight, sound, taste) to calm the nervous system during emotional pain.

IMPROVE the Moment

Imagery, Meaning, Prayer, Relaxation, One Thing in the moment, brief Vacation, Encouragement—micro-practices for surviving distress.

Crisis Survival Skills

Tools for navigating moments of intense overwhelm without making things worse.

EMOTION REGULATION SKILLS

Understanding the Purpose of Emotions

Emotions communicate needs, motivate action, and signal what matters. They are meaningful, not failures.

Labeling Emotions

Identifying feelings with clarity ("I feel betrayed," "I feel anxious"). Doing so reduces intensity and brings structure to chaos.

Opposite Action

Acting opposite to an unhelpful emotional urge (e.g., staying when you want to run, softening when you want to lash out).

Checking the Facts

Assessing whether an emotion fits the situation or is being amplified by past pain, assumptions, or fears.

ABC PLEASE (Reducing Vulnerability)

Daily practices that keep emotional capacity strong:

- **A**ctivities
- **B**uild Mastery
- **C**ope Ahead
- **PLEASE**: Physical health, balanced eating, avoiding substances, sleep, exercise.

Build Mastery

Doing small, consistent actions that grow competency and confidence.

INTERPERSONAL EFFECTIVENESS SKILLS

DEAR MAN (Objective Effectiveness)

A communication structure for asking for what you need clearly and respectfully:

Describe, Express, Assert, Reinforce, Mindfully, Appear confident, Negotiate.

GIVE (Relationship Effectiveness)

Gentle, Interested, Validate, Easy manner—skills for maintaining connection with warmth and respect.

FAST (Self-Respect Effectiveness)

Fair, no Apologies for values, Stick to truth, Truthful—skills for honoring one's identity and boundaries.

Validation (Six Levels)

Communicating to someone that their experience "makes sense" based on causes, history, or context—even when you disagree.

Walking the Middle Path

Balancing acceptance and change. Holding tension without swinging to extremes.

Co-regulation

Regulating emotions through connection with another person. In Christian language: communion, fellowship, shared presence.

DBT Terms and Their Spiritual Parallels

(Adapted from the foundational work of Dr. Marsha Linehan, developer of Dialectical Behavioral Therapy, 1993, and reinterpreted through biblical theology and the Mind-Spirit Bible Practice framework.)

Dialectical Behavioral Therapy (DBT)

DBT is a behavioral model created by psychologist Dr. Marsha Linehan to help individuals regulate emotions, improve relationships, and endure distress without self-destructive behavior. The term *dialectical* means that two seemingly opposing truths can coexist—for example, *I accept myself as I am, and I am also called to change.*

Spiritual Integration:

In this book, DBT is interpreted through the biblical principle of divine dialectic—where the Holy Spirit integrates grace and truth, emotion and wisdom, justice and mercy. The Spirit brings unity where the world divides. As John 1:17 says, ". . . grace and truth came through Jesus Christ" (ESV).

Mind States and Their Biblical Parallels

DBT Concept	Definition	Spiritual Parallel	Example Skill	Scriptural Anchor
Emotion Mind → The Mind of the Flesh	A state where emotion dominates thought and behavior; feelings are treated as facts.	Paul's "mind governed by the flesh" (Romans 8:6)—reactive, impulsive, and self-protective.	Observing and describing emotions without judgment.	"Be still and know that I am God." (Psalm 46:10)

DBT Concept	Definition	Spiritual Parallel	Example Skill	Scriptural Anchor
Reason Mind → The Mind of the World	A logical, analytical state that suppresses emotion; intellect without grace.	"Knowledge puffs up, but love builds up." (1 Corinthians 8:1)	Checking the facts and using logic with compassion.	"Trust in the Lord . . . lean not on your own understanding." (Proverbs 3:5)
Wise Mind → The Mind of the Spirit	The integration of emotion and reason—calm awareness guided by truth and love.	"The mind governed by the Spirit is life and peace." (Romans 8:6)	Mindfulness and prayerful reflection.	"The peace of God . . . will guard your hearts and minds in Christ Jesus." (Philippians 4:7)

Core DBT Skills and Their Biblical Counterparts

DBT Skill	Purpose	Spiritual Reflection	Example Scripture
Mindfulness	To stay aware of the present moment without judgment.	Remaining aware of God's presence and observing thought and emotion as they are.	"Pause in His presence."—*Psalm 62:8*
Distress Tolerance	To endure pain skillfully without acting impulsively or destructively.	Faith in suffering—learning to wait and trust in the wilderness.	"Though I sit in darkness, the Lord will be my light."—*Micah 7:8*
Emotion Regulation	To understand, name, and manage emotions rather than be ruled by them.	Allowing the Spirit to govern emotion, transforming reactivity into peace.	"The Spirit gives us power, love, and self-control."—*2 Timothy 1:7*

DBT Skill	Purpose	Spiritual Reflection	Example Scripture
Interpersonal Effectiveness	To communicate needs and maintain relationships with integrity.	Speaking the truth in love; balancing honesty with grace.	"Speak the truth in love."— *Ephesians 4:15*

Dialectical Thinking—The Paradox of Grace and Truth

DBT Definition:

Holding two truths at once—acceptance and change, emotion and logic, self-compassion and accountability.

Spiritual Parallel:

The divine paradox of Jesus—fully human and fully God. In Him, truth and tenderness, justice and mercy, meet in perfect harmony. As Psalm 85:10 says, ". . . righteousness and peace kiss each other."

Sin and Disconnection

DBT View: Emotional dysregulation and impulsivity often arise when we seek relief apart from mindful awareness.

Spiritual View: Sin is misalignment with God's Spirit—acting or not acting in ways that disconnect us from divine presence and peace.

The *Mind of the Flesh* seeks false comfort.
The *Mind of the World* seeks control.
The *Mind of the Spirit* seeks communion.

Through repentance (spiritual mindfulness) we return to alignment, allowing the Spirit's peace to refill the void. "Let anyone who is thirsty come to Me and drink . . . rivers of living water will flow from within them" (John 7:37–38).

DBT Skill Sets as Spiritual Disciplines

DBT Skill Category	Spiritual Discipline	Description
Mindfulness	Prayerful awareness	Staying conscious of God in the moment.
Distress Tolerance	Surrender and endurance	Bearing suffering with faith and trust.
Emotion Regulation	Self-examination and surrender	Identifying and offering emotions to God for transformation.

DBT Skill Category	Spiritual Discipline	Description
Interpersonal Effectiveness	Confession and reconciliation	Pursuing truth, grace, and unity in relationships.

Summary Table—The Four Spiritual Practices of the Mind–Spirit Bible Practice

DBT Skill	Biblical Parallel	Spiritual Outcome
Mindfulness	The Mind of the Spirit	Awareness of God's presence.
Distress Tolerance	Sitting in the Wilderness	Endurance through surrender.
Emotion Regulation	Letting the Spirit Rule the Heart	Peace and inner alignment.
Interpersonal Effectiveness	Speaking the Truth in Love	Reconciliation and integrity.

DBT in the Context of Community: How Each Skill Sustains the Body of Christ

DBT Skill	Spiritual Parallel	How It Sustains the Body of Christ	Scriptural Reflection
Mindfulness	Awareness of God's presence	Keeps the Church awake to the movement of the Spirit; helps us listen before reacting.	"Be still, and know that I am God."—Psalm 46:10

DBT Skill	Spiritual Parallel	How It Sustains the Body of Christ	Scriptural Reflection
Distress Tolerance	Persevering love / Long-suffering	Enables us to stay at the table when community feels messy; prevents rupture from becoming division.	"Bear with one another in love."—Ephesians 4:2
Emotion Regulation	Peace that surpasses understanding	Calms the collective nervous system of the Church; allows peace to rule in our hearts and relationships.	"Let the peace of Christ rule in your hearts."—Colossians 3:15
Interpersonal Effectiveness	Speaking truth in love / Graceful boundaries	Builds trust and mutual respect; makes correction and collaboration redemptive rather than reactive.	"Speak the truth in love, growing in every way more like Christ."—Ephesians 4:15

DBT Skill	Spiritual Parallel	How It Sustains the Body of Christ	Scriptural Reflection
Walking the Middle Path	Grace + Growth / Mercy + Truth	Balances acceptance and change in relationships; models discipleship that is patient yet transformative.	"Mercy and truth have met together; righteousness and peace have kissed."—Psalm 85:10
Radical Acceptance	Surrender to God's will	Frees us from resisting reality; allows the Church to grieve, forgive, and move forward together.	"Not my will, but Yours be done."—Luke 22:42

The Origins and Legacy of Dialectical Behavior Therapy (DBT)

1. The Story of Dr. Marsha Linehan

Dr. Marsha M. Linehan, Ph.D., is a clinical psychologist and professor emerita at the University of Washington. In the 1970s and 1980s, she began working with patients who struggled with chronic suicidal behavior and what was then diagnosed as Borderline Personality Disorder (BPD). At that time, no empirically supported treatment existed for these individuals—many clinicians even considered them "untreatable."

Drawing from her background in behavioral psychology, cognitive therapy, and mindfulness, Dr. Linehan developed what became Dialectical Behavior Therapy (DBT)—a treatment that integrates both acceptance and change. The term *dialectical* refers to the synthesis of opposites: holding two seemingly opposing truths at once (for example, "I am doing the best I can" and "I need to try harder").

In her memoir *Building a Life Worth Living*, Linehan (2020) revealed publicly for the first time that she herself had been hospitalized as a young woman for extreme emotional suffering and self-harm. This disclosure reframed DBT not only as a scientific innovation but also as an act of deep compassion born from lived experience. As she said in a separate interview, "I developed DBT to treat the most miserable people I could find—and I was one of them" (Carey 2011).

2. Core Elements of DBT

DBT blends strategies from several traditions:

- Cognitive Behavioral Therapy (CBT): Identifying and changing unhelpful thoughts and behaviors.

- Mindfulness (from Zen and contemplative practice): Developing nonjudgmental awareness of the present moment.

- Dialectical philosophy: Learning to balance acceptance with change.

- Skills training: Building four primary skill sets—Mindfulness, Distress Tolerance, Emotion Regulation, and Interpersonal Effectiveness.

These skills are now used far beyond their original population. DBT has demonstrated efficacy in treating depression, anxiety, eating disorders, post-traumatic stress, substance use disorders, and emotional dysregulation in both adults and adolescents (Linehan et al. 2015; Swales 2016; Lynch et al. 2007).

3. DBT in Today's World

DBT is now considered one of the most evidence-based treatments for emotion dysregulation worldwide. Its use has expanded across clinical, correctional, educational, and community settings. Modern DBT programs often integrate spiritual, cultural, and trauma-informed adaptations, reflecting Linehan's original vision that therapy must be both scientifically sound and deeply humane.

As Dr. Linehan often emphasized, DBT is not just a therapy—it's a way of life, built on the commitment to create a *"life worth living."*

Connect With
The Author

This book was never meant to end at the final page.

The Mind–Spirit Bible Practice was written as a companion—a way of learning to live from the Mind of the Spirit in real time, with real emotions, real relationships, and a real God who meets us in the gap. If these pages stirred something in you—clarity, conviction, relief, or even discomfort—you are not meant to carry that alone.

I created Mind–Spirit Bible Practice (MSB) as an ongoing space for integration at the intersection of faith, emotional health, and embodied discipleship. It exists for those who long to follow Jesus with their whole selves—mind, body, and spirit—without shame, spiritual bypassing, or fragmentation.

You can learn more about the MSB framework, access additional resources, and continue this practice at:

www.msbpractice.com

If you'd like to reach out, share how this book met you, or inquire about resources, you can contact me at:

info@msbpractice.com

You can also find ongoing reflections, teachings, and community conversations on social media:

@mindspiritbiblepractice

My prayer is that this work continues to help you notice God's presence more readily, respond more gently to yourself and others, and trust the Spirit's work of integration over time. Healing is not a destination—it is a way of walking with God.

Thank you for letting this book walk with you for a while.

— Nicole Doña

References

Bishop, Scott R., Mark Lau, Shauna Shapiro, Linda Carlson, Nicholas D. Anderson, James Carmody, Zindel V. Segal, Susan Abbey, Michael Speca, Drew Velting, and Gerald Devins. "Mindfulness: A Proposed Operational Definition." *Clinical Psychology: Science and Practice* 11, no. 3 (2004): 230–241. https://doi.org/10.1093/clipsy.bph077.

Carey, Benedict. "Expert on Mental Illness Reveals Her Own Fight." *The New York Times*, June 23, 2011. https://www.nytimes.com/2011/06/23/health/23lives.html.

Fruzzetti, Alan E. "DBT with Families." In *Dialectical Behavior Therapy in Clinical Practice: Applications across Disorders and Settings*, edited by Thomas A. Dimeff and Kelly Koerner. New York: Guilford Press, 2007.

Gratz, Kim L., and Lizabeth Roemer. "Multidimensional Assessment of Emotion Regulation and Dysregulation: Development, Factor Structure, and Initial Validation of the Difficulties in Emotion Regulation Scale." *Journal of Psychopathology and Behavioral Assessment* 26, no. 1 (2004): 41–54. https://doi.org/10.1023/B:JOBA.0000007455.08539.94.

Hayes, Steven C., Kirk D. Strosahl, and Kelly G. Wilson. *Acceptance and Commitment Therapy: An Experiential Approach to Behavior Change*. New York: Guilford Press, 1999.

Hayes, Steven C., Kirk D. Strosahl, and Kelly G. Wilson. *Acceptance and Commitment Therapy, Second Edition: The Process and Practice of Mindful Change*. New York: Guilford Press, 2011.

Kabat-Zinn, Jon. *Wherever You Go, There You Are: Mindfulness Meditation in Everyday Life*. New York: Hyperion, 1994.

Koerner, Kelly. *Doing Dialectical Behavior Therapy: A Practical Guide*. New York: The Guilford Press, 2012.

Kristeller, Jean L. "Mindfulness, Wisdom, and Eating: Applying a Multi-Domain Model of Meditation Effects." *Constructivism in the Human Sciences* 8, no. 2 (2003): 107–118.

Linehan, Marsha M. *Cognitive-Behavioral Treatment of Borderline Personality Disorder*. New York: Guilford Press, 1993.

Linehan, Marsha M. *Skills Training Manual for Treating Borderline Personality Disorder*. New York: The Guilford Press, 1993.

Linehan, Marsha M. *DBT Skills Training Manual*. 2nd ed. New York: Guilford Press, 2015.

Linehan, Marsha M. *Building a Life Worth Living: A Memoir*. New York: Random House, 2020.

Lynch, Thomas R. *The Skills Training Manual for Radically Open Dialectical Behavior Therapy: A Clinician's Guide for Treating Disorders of Overcontrol*. Oakland, CA: New Harbinger Publications, 2018.

Lynch, Thomas R., William T. Trost, Nicholas Salsman, and Marsha M. Linehan. "Dialectical Behavior Therapy for Borderline Personality Disorder." *Annual Review of Clinical Psychology* 3 (2007): 181–205. https://doi.org/10.1146/annurev.clinpsy.2.022305.095229.

Neacsiu, Andrada D., Shireen L. Rizvi, and Marsha M. Linehan. "Dialectical Behavior Therapy Skills Use as a Mediator and Outcome of Treatment for Borderline Personality Disorder." *Behaviour Research and Therapy* 48, no. 9 (2010): 832–839. https://doi.org/10.1016/j.brat.2010.05.017.

Robins, Clive J. "Zen Principles and Mindfulness Practice in Dialectical Behavior Therapy." *Cognitive and Behavioral Practice* 9, no. 1 (2002): 50–57. https://doi.org/10.1016/S1077-7229(02)80040-2.

Siegel, Daniel J. *The Developing Mind: How Relationships and the Brain Interact to Shape Who We Are.* 2nd ed. New York: Guilford Press, 2012.

Soler, Joaquim, José Carlos Pascual, Teresa Tiana, et al. "Dialectical Behaviour Therapy Skills Training Compared to Standard Group Therapy in Borderline Personality Disorder: A 3-Month Randomised Controlled Clinical Trial." *Behaviour Research and Therapy* 47, no. 5 (2009): 353–358. https://doi.org/10.1016/j.brat.2009.01.013.

Stoffers-Winterling, Jutta M., Birgit A. Völlm, Gerta Rücker, Antje Timmer, Nick Huband, and Klaus Lieb. "Psychological Therapies for People with Borderline Personality Disorder." *Cochrane Database of Systematic Reviews* (2012), no. 8: CD005652. https://doi.org/10.1002/14651858.CD005652.pub2.

Swales, Michaela A., ed. *The Oxford Handbook of Dialectical Behaviour Therapy.* Oxford: Oxford University Press, 2016.

Willard, Dallas. *The Spirit of the Disciplines: Understanding How God Changes Lives.* San Francisco: HarperOne, 1998.

Wright, N. T. *Simply Jesus: A New Vision of Who He Was, What He Did, and Why He Matters.* New York: HarperOne, 2012.

About the Author

Nicole Doña is a Christian author, nonprofit founder, and mental-health advocate passionate about integrating faith and psychology for emotional healing. She is the author of *The Mind-Spirit Bible Practice*— a groundbreaking guide that bridges Scripture and Dialectical Behavior Therapy (DBT) to bring emotional and spiritual wholeness to believ- 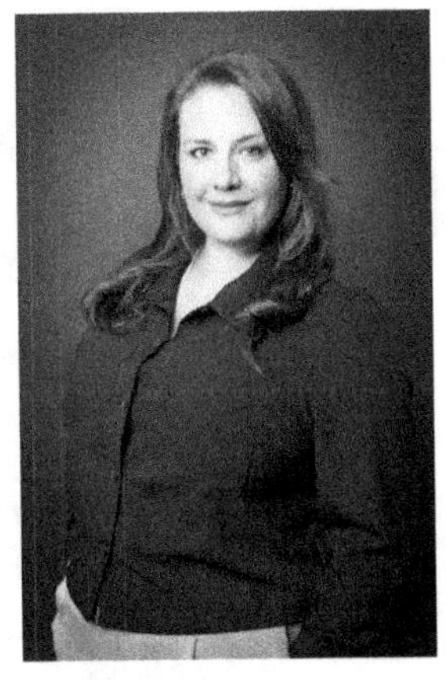 ers, clinicians, and ministries alike. A brain tumor survivor, wife, and foster mom, Nicole writes from lived experience, weaving neuroscience, trauma recovery, and biblical wisdom into a practical framework for transformation. She has led policy reforms in San Francisco for system-involved youth, advanced statewide mental-health reforms across California, and collaborated with global brain-health leaders through the University of California, San Francisco. In 2015, she received a Certificate of Honor from the San Francisco City & County Board of Supervisors for her contributions to mental-health policy and advocacy. She lives in the San Francisco Bay Area with her husband, Josh.